SLEEP
AND ITS
DISORDERS

WHAT YOU SHOULD KNOW

Robert G. Hooper, M.D.

Illustrations and Graphs, Melissa Mulera

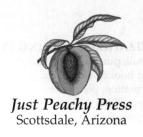

Just Peachy Press
Scottsdale, Arizona

Although the author and publisher have exhaustively researched all sources to ensure the accuracy and completeness of the information contained in this book, we assume no responsibility for errors, inaccuracies, omissions or any inconsistency herein. Any slights of people or organizations are unintentional. Readers should use their own judgment or consult a medical expert or their personal physicians for specific applications to their individual problems.

Illustrations and Graphs by Melissa Mulera
Desktop Publishing Services by C² Computer Creations

First printing 2001

ISBN: 0-9700026-4-5

LCCN: 00-091160

SLEEP
AND ITS
DISORDERS

WHAT YOU SHOULD KNOW

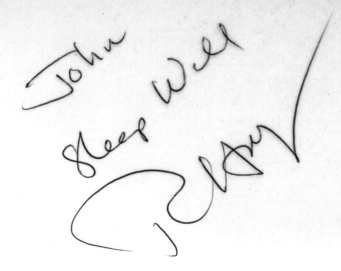

John
Sleep Well

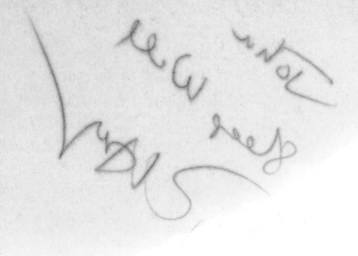

ACKNOWLEDGMENTS

The preparation of this book has taken time and effort from many people. They provided encouragement, support, reviews, criticism, proofreading, technical advice, and illustrations. My wife, Dana, has performed most of these roles at one time or another. She has been the person who makes my words work, if they do to any extent. Without a doubt, another person who contributed greatly to this volume was Lorraine Fischer at C^2 Computer Creations in Scottsdale, Arizona. For her efforts, I cannot thank her adequately. She has been a great partner in this project. Melissa Mulera's illustrations speak for themselves. There would be no book without them.

Many thanks belong to my staff, my partners, the staff at the Scottsdale Healthcare Shea, Sleep Disorder Center, my friends and my family for their encouragement and reviews of the book.

ACKNOWLEDGMENTS

The preparation of this book has taken time and effort from many people. They provided encouragement, support, reviews, criticism, proofreading, technical advice, and illustrations. My wife, Dana, has performed most of these roles at one time or another. She has been the person who makes my words work, if they do to any extent. Without a doubt, another person who contributed greatly to this volume was Lorraine Fischer at C Computer Creations in Scottsdale, Arizona. For her efforts, I cannot thank her adequately. She has been a great partner in this project. Melissa Mutera's illustrations speak for themselves. There would be no book without them. Many thanks belong to my staff, my partners, the staff at the Scottsdale Healthcare Shea, Sleep Disorder Center, my friends and my family for their encouragement and reviews of the book.

TABLE OF CONTENTS

Section III: Sleep Apnea Syndrome

Section IV: Common Sleep Problems and Disorders

LIST OF TABLES AND FIGURES

PREFACE

Early in my career as a physician, I served in the United States Army and was Chief of the Pulmonary Function Laboratories at Walter Reed Army Medical Center in Washington, D.C. Soon after assuming my responsibilities, I was asked to see and help with the evaluation of a twenty-year-old soldier who kept falling asleep while driving. He had been observed while sleeping to have terrible snoring and choking spells. He was suffering from what was then a recently described medical problem called sleep apnea.

Now a quarter of a century later, sleep apnea has become recognized as one of the major health problems of our country, affecting more than four percent of the population. Information about the problems of sleep has grown rapidly and techniques to evaluate sleep and its problems have been developed. Special laboratories and sleep centers have been created where physicians with special knowledge of sleep disorders perform tests for them. Despite the growth in knowledge and technologies, communicating what we know to people who have a problem is difficult.

In practicing sleep medicine, I daily have to explain sleep problems and their treatments to people who suffer from them. A few problems are common and account for the majority of those that physicians treat, but there

are many sleep disorders. This book developed from my
years of describing these disorders to my patients and my
desire to have a book they could use with this basic information on sleep and sleep disorders. It concentrates on
the common problems and provides an introduction to
sleep, sleep testing, and what a patient should know about
frequent sleep disorders.

INTRODUCTION

Sleep and mankind cannot be separated. Throughout our lives, sleep is an essential part of each day. One-third of our lifetime, fully 20 to 25 years, is spent asleep. It is not surprising that we are all interested in sleep. Did we sleep well last night? Did we sleep enough? How did we feel this morning?

Sleep Medicine, as a field, has been growing rapidly over the past 20 years. Our understanding of sleep problems and the sleep disorders increases each year. Also, our ability to help with the problems and treat the disorders has increased tremendously over this period of time.

It is helpful for someone interested or concerned about sleep to know about normal sleep and the disorders which can affect it. This book was prepared to help you understand sleep and how to approach sleep problems.

The fact that you are reading this sentence suggests you have an interest in sleep and its disorders. This book provides information that may improve your understanding of sleep and assist you in helping yourself or your loved ones with a sleep problem. The goal of presenting an overview of the knowledge of normal sleep and sleep related problems allows a reader to become better informed.

As you look at the contents, you will notice that the book has been organized into sections, each of which has a common purpose. The first sections present general information about sleep and the evaluation and testing for sleep problems. Later sections present information on the types of sleep problems and how we classify them. Specific types of problems are then reviewed to provide more detailed information about them. Lastly, the appendix provides a glossary of terms, some self-help ideas and a sleep diary for your use.

You may want to read from beginning to end, or if you have a specific interest, you can go directly to that section. Regardless of your approach, you will, hopefully, find useful information. Please remember, sleep related symptoms may be the presenting feature of a serious medical problem. This book should serve as an aid for answering your questions about sleep. Consult a professional such as your physician or a sleep specialist for medical advice.

"To sleep: Perchance to dream: Ay there's the rub;"

Hamlet, Act III, Scene I

SLEEP AND
ITS EVALUATION

To understand problems with sleep, it is necessary to have a knowledge of normal sleep and how it is tested and measured. This section will help you understand sleep.

Chapter 1 - Normal Sleep

Chapter 2 - Sleep and Its Evaluation

SECTION I

SLEEP AND
ITS EVALUATION

To understand problems with sleep, it is necessary to have a knowledge of normal sleep and how it is tested and measured. This section will help you understand sleep.

Chapter 1 - Normal Sleep

Chapter 2 - Sleep and Its Evaluation

Chapter One

Normal Sleep

WHY DO WE SLEEP?

We need sleep. We sleep because we cannot go without it. We must sleep, but why? Actually no one knows why we must sleep. A great deal is known about sleep - when, how, how much, and what happens during sleep - but why we sleep is not known.

There are theories about why we must sleep. Two theories are currently thought to be the most likely explanations. One is that sleep is needed to conserve our energies. Our metabolic processes need time to rest themselves for the coming day.

The second theory is that sleep is required to restore our bodies. It suggests that sleep gives our bodies time to catch up, time to repair metabolic processes, and time to replace essential metabolic building blocks. This second theory, the need for time to restore our bodies, seems to make the most sense in view of current knowledge.

Whatever the reason, we all sleep. Everyone. More or less, better or worse, sleep is an essential part of our lives.

NORMAL SLEEP

What is normal sleep? Normal sleep is obvious to us all. It is what we have those special nights, those nights when we awake in the morning relaxed, refreshed and re-energized. A good night's sleep is just that. But how do we put that into words or some measure so that we can compare sleep from different nights and different people?

We can define sleep in several ways. From the sleeper's point of view, how long you sleep (its duration), when you sleep (the time of day), and how you feel when you wake up (its effect), are obviously very important. From the view of the sleeper's physiology, many facts may be recorded to measure sleep. The facts include changes in brain waves, muscular tone, respirations, and cardiac events.

HOW LONG DO WE SLEEP?

How much sleep is normal? The obvious answer to this is "enough" sleep - an adequate amount. However, enough sleep varies considerably from person to person. For normal individuals, adequate sleep varies from 5 - 12 hours a night. The average is very close to the 8 hours that all of us have heard about from the time of our childhood. However, 20% of mankind does nicely on less than seven hours, while another 20% needs more than 9 hours to have an adequate sleep.

The amount of time we sleep varies. From day to day and week to week, many factors affect the duration of our sleep. Work demands, social events, and family matters all affect the length of our sleep on a specific night. While we can vary the time we sleep, the duration of sleep needed to be refreshed stays fairly constant. The sleep we require is greatest when we are infants and decreases as we grow older.

What then, is the normal amount of sleep for you? Only you can answer the question for yourself. If you sleep 8 hours a night and you usually awake comfortable and refreshed, then 8 hours is the normal amount of sleep for you. If you are one of those fortunate people who only require 6 or 7 hours for the same feelings, then that is a normal amount of sleep for you. In addition, you have gained an extra one or more hours a day to enjoy.

A change in sleep duration is the most frequent problem with sleep that someone will notice. If you have recently changed the amount of sleep that you are getting from shorter to longer, or longer to shorter, this change may signify problems.

WHEN DO WE SLEEP?

The period of the day when sleep occurs can vary. For most of us, sleep begins between the hours of 9 and 12 P.M. and lasts till 5 to 8 A.M. The timing of sleep, like the duration of sleep, varies widely among individuals.

Of course, modern mankind can choose when we sleep just as we can choose how long we sleep. Sleep can be put off. Coffee, soda, or tea (caffeine) can be ingested. Lights can brighten our nights and shades can make our days like night. We can choose when to wake up. Alarm clocks have become a central part of many of our mornings. Changing the time allowed for sleep may be caused by personal activities, work responsibilities, illness, and social disruptions.

Beside these man-made reasons, there is a natural tendency for a preferred time to sleep. We have to sleep and our body tells us when it is time for us to sleep. The circadian rhythm is one reason for variation in when we sleep. The rhythm is the internal biological clock that regulates many of our body's functions. It is a clock that runs on a 24-hour schedule, for most of us. The circadian rhythm tells our bodies when they should sleep. There are individuals who have shorter and longer cycles. They have different needs for sleep and will sleep at the time the clock tells them to sleep.

The circadian rhythm is set and regulated by the light reaching our brains through our eyes. The result is that most people, and their circadian rhythms, prefer sleep to occur at night.

The other driving force determining when we sleep could be called the 'Exhaustion' effect. The amount of sleep the night before and the day's activities will contribute to the need for sleep.

THE STAGES OF SLEEP

Physicians and physiologists are able to view sleep differently. They are able to understand and analyze tests of respiration, muscle, and brain function during sleep.

Normal sleep has physiologic patterns which can be measured with appropriate instruments. Distinctive patterns have been defined and are called the "stages" of sleep. Sleep stages are determined by brain wave (electroencephalogram - EEG) and muscle tone (electromyogram - EMG) measurements. The overall pattern of sleep stages during a night is called sleep architecture.

The EEG and EMG allow us to separate sleep into 5 distinct stages; stages 1 through 4 are known as non-REM sleep and the 5th stage is called REM (Rapid Eye Movement) sleep. A normal night of sleep will demonstrate all of these stages in varying degrees. It is not an orderly progression of stages - 1, 2, 3, 4, REM and then back - rather it changes irregularly during the night with Stage 2 being the focal point of sleep. Adequate amounts of all stages of sleep are obtained with normal sleep. Abnormalities in sleep architecture frequently can be noted with sleep disorders.

SLEEP STAGES

STAGE I - LIGHT SLEEP
➤ Entry stage for sleep
➤ Person awakes easily and may be aware of surroundings

STAGE II - MODERATE SLEEP
➤ Focal point of sleep
➤ Majority of sleep time spent in this stage

STAGES III & IV - DEEP SLEEP
➤ Time in these stages is needed to feel rested on awakening.

STAGE REM - RAPID EYE MOVEMENT SLEEP
➤ Muscles are totally relaxed in REM sleep.
➤ The closed eyes move rapidly.
➤ Brain waves are the same as while awake.
➤ This is the sleep stage where most dreams occur.

It is convenient to think of sleep in terms of depth. When we awake from sleep sometimes it is so sound, so deep, it is hard to wake up. Most everyone has experienced the feeling. The sleep stages may be thought of as progressing from lighter to deeper with stage one being the lightest and stage four the deepest.

REM (Rapid Eye Movement) sleep is an interesting stage of sleep. It has also been referred to as "Dream Sleep." When someone is awakened from REM sleep, they usually report they were dreaming at the time. Dreams occur in other sleep stages, but not as frequently.

REM sleep is also interesting because of the physiologic changes noted when it is present. During REM sleep the pattern of events recorded are the same as seen while awake. There are two major differences. The person in REM sleep is totally relaxed with no muscle movements of any kind. During wakefulness and the other stages of sleep, sensitive measurements by the EMG demonstrate activity in muscles. The second difference seen in REM sleep is the rapid movement of the eyes with the lids closed.

Examples of the importance of sleep stages are Stages 3 and 4. These stages are known as slow wave sleep, because of a characteristic EEG pattern showing slow brain waves. These deeper stages seem to be very important for the restorative qualities of sleep. If the time spent in stages 3 and 4 sleep is too short, then no matter how much time is spent asleep, an individual will feel sleepy and unrefreshed after a night of sleep.

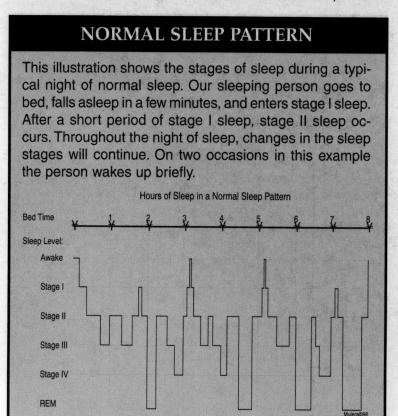

NORMAL SLEEP PATTERN

This illustration shows the stages of sleep during a typical night of normal sleep. Our sleeping person goes to bed, falls asleep in a few minutes, and enters stage I sleep. After a short period of stage I sleep, stage II sleep occurs. Throughout the night of sleep, changes in the sleep stages will continue. On two occasions in this example the person wakes up briefly.

Hours of Sleep in a Normal Sleep Pattern

Figure 1-1

During a night of sleep, all stages of sleep occur. Instead of an orderly progression, sleep moves to different stages randomly with stage II being the center of sleep. There are expected patterns and an example is seen in the accompanying figure.

Sleep architecture changes with age. The elderly have far different patterns from those of infants. These changes are fairly predictable and reproducible. It is the measurement of the EEG and EMG during sleep that allows the physician to estimate the quality and quantity of the time spent in various stages of sleep.

CHANGES IN SLEEP STAGES WITH AGE

As we age, our sleep changes. An older person needs less time asleep than a younger one. Most of the change is seen as a reduction in stage III and IV sleep (deep sleep).

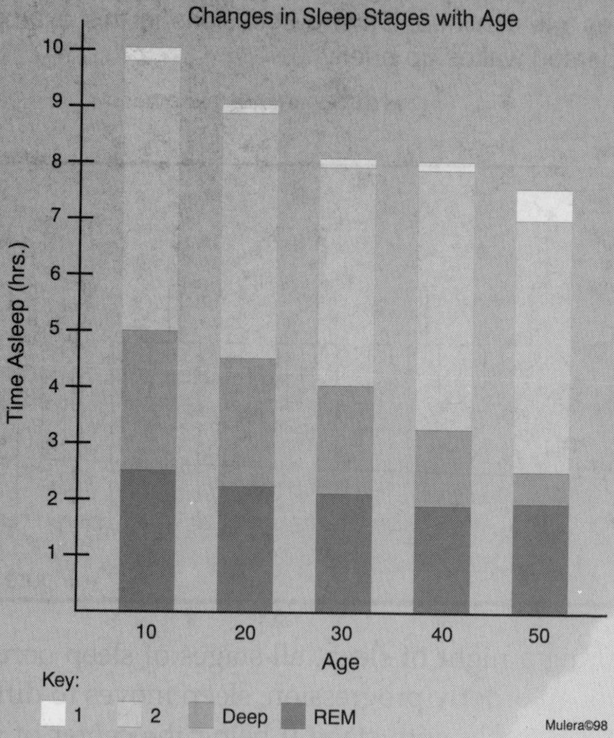

Changes in Sleep Stages with Age

Key:
1 · 2 · Deep · REM

Mulera©98

Figure 1-2

Normal Sleep
CHAPTER SUMMARY

WHY WE SLEEP
- To rest our bodies
- To rebuild our metabolic functions

NORMAL SLEEP
- Duration needed to feel rested
- The time of day we sleep
- Physiologic changes

HOW LONG DO WE SLEEP?
- Duration needed to feel rested
  - Ranges from 5 to 12 hours
  - Average 8 hours
  - Individual needs
- Circadian Rhythm controls
- Behavior and habits alter

WHEN DO WE SLEEP?
- A regular schedule
- Guided by the Circadian Rhythm
- Controlled by light
- Nighttime preferred

SLEEP PHYSIOLOGY
- Stages of sleep
  - Lighter - Stages I and II
  - Deeper - Stages III and IV
    - Needed for restful night of sleep
- Pattern of stages predictable
- Pattern changes with age

Chapter Two

Sleep and
Its Evaluation

THE EVALUATION
OF SLEEP PROBLEMS

Do you, a family member, or a friend have a sleep problem? If so, where should you start and what should you do? Common sense should be followed. Most problems with sleep are not urgent and it is safe to allow time to work on the problem. Books and brochures can be of help. Libraries, book stores, newspaper articles and the Internet contain useful information. Frequently, friends or family members can provide some help.

It is possible, after learning a little about sleep, to find that no problem exists. Or, general information about sleep may give you enough insight to help clear up the problem.

Frequently, just beginning regular sleep habits that promote quality sleep can solve many sleep complaints. There are many lists of tips for sleeping which can be used. My version of "Hints for a Good Night's Sleep" is reproduced in the appendix.

There are simple tools which may be used to measure sleep that can help in your self-assessment. You can use the Epworth Sleepiness Scale to help you judge if you are too sleepy. It is reproduced in the appendix of this book. If you have the equipment, a tape recording of an hour of your sleep can be helpful. Even more dramatic would be a video of your sleep. A sleep diary, a recording of your daily activities and sleep, may be requested by a physician. Completing a sleep diary before you seek professional help might aid you in identifying what is happening with your sleep. A sample is in the appendix.

Advice can be sought from a professional. A physician can usually give you sound advice and directions on how to solve any problems you may be having with sleep. There are physicians with considerable experience and training in sleep disorders. Your physician may ask you to see one of these sleep specialists, or you may seek out a specialist on your own.

A sleep specialist has had extra training and experience with the medical problems of sleep. Most sleep specialists were originally trained in another field of medicine and frequently practice both sleep medicine and their primary field of training. Pulmonologists (specialists in lung disease) commonly become specialists in sleep because of the number of patients with breathing problems during sleep. Neurologists (specialists in diseases of the nervous system) have become sleep specialists because of their association with disturbed levels of consciousness and narcolepsy. Psychiatrists (specialists in behavioral and psychiatric disorders) have become interested in sleep because of the association of sleep disorders with their primary field of interest. Likewise, otolaryngologists (ear, nose and throat specialists) have become interested in sleep because of the benefit of certain surgical procedures they perform in the treatment of patients with sleep disorders.

When you first visit a physician about a sleep problem, he will begin an evaluation that is common to all medical problems. First, a history of the events surrounding your symptoms or complaints will be obtained. The history helps to identify the problem and forms a list of possible causes - a differential diagnosis. A physical examination will be performed and laboratory studies may be ordered to support the suspected diagnosis or to rule out other diagnoses.

SLEEP HISTORY

When trying to help someone with a sleep problem, it is important for the physician to know all the events that may affect someone's sleep. Consequently, many questions must be asked.

Events beginning with the time you go to bed until the time you get up are important because they describe the characteristics of your sleep pattern. It is important to know what the patient and his bedmate have observed about the patient's sleep. Does the patient snore, awake during the night, thrash during sleep, or require a long time to go to sleep?

Daytime activities have a significant effect on sleep. It is important to know what happens on an average day, including medications taken, caffeine products used, naps taken, and activities performed during the day. This picture of an average day is important in analyzing sleep problems since many activities and habits can affect the quality of sleep.

Occasionally, you will be asked to keep a sleep diary. A diary of both day and nighttime events can help the physician analyze your sleep problems. Often this allows you to identify and understand how to change your behavior and help sleep-related symptoms. An example can be found in the appendix of this book.

SLEEP STUDY (POLYSOMNOGRAM)

A polysomnogram is a study of sleep. It records and analyzes the physiologic events that occur during a night of sleep. Polysomnograms have been widely available only since 1980. It is the major tool used in the diagnosis and treatment of patients with sleep disorders.

What should be expected when having a polysomnogram? The studies are scheduled at bedtime hours when most individuals will be at their maximum sleepiness. The study lasts all night with the goal of observing a full night of sleep. To achieve this, they are carried out in quiet comfortable rooms that are more like hotel rooms than hospital rooms.

Since the measurement of the physiologic events during sleep is the purpose of the test, a number of painless monitors must be used. These are applied to the skin with adhesive or worn connected with straps. The things monitored include; brain waves, muscle movement (chin, eyes, legs), air movement (nose and mouth), chest and abdominal movement, electrocardiogram (ECG), and the oxygen levels in the arterial blood.

During the study, the brain waves will be monitored with an electroencephalogram (EEG). Small electrode leads similar to those used for an electrocardiogram will

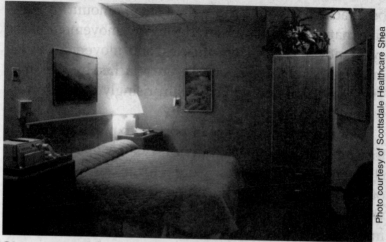

Photo courtesy of Scottsdale Healthcare Shea

Sleep laboratory bedroom. This photo shows a typical room in a sleep laboratory. Effort is made to have the room comfortable and similar to a typical bedroom. A careful observer will note the monitoring equipment on the bedside table and hanging on the wall opposite the bed.

Figure 2-1

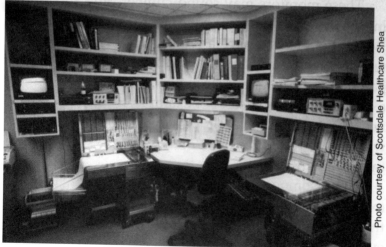

Photo courtesy of Scottsdale Healthcare Shea

Sleep laboratory monitoring area. While a patient sleeps in the bedroom, technicians monitor the person and his physiologic variables on equipment in the monitoring area.

Figure 2-2

be attached to your head with a small amount of adhesive material. Similar electrodes record movement of the eyes, movement of chin muscles, and movement of leg muscles. All of these electrodes are attached by adhesive. They are small and will have surprisingly little effect on the ability to sleep.

For the study, it is very important to measure respiratory and cardiac events. Monitors will be attached to the chest and abdominal wall in order to measure movements of these muscles while breathing. It is important to know whether air is moving through the nose or mouth. To make these types of measurements, a small plastic tube will be worn under the nose. And lastly, in order to measure oxygenation during sleep, a tape or clip with a light sensor in it will be wrapped around a finger, a toe, or an earlobe during the night. All of these monitors will be recording the events of sleep throughout the night.

These monitors may sound cumbersome and irritating, however, most people have no problem falling asleep. While it is great to have a typical night of sleep during testing, much important information can be obtained regardless. A full night of sleep is not required to make or exclude most diagnoses. For example, if severe sleep apnea is present on the early portion of a study, the study will be stopped so that a form of treatment may be tried that same night.

A polysomnogram study is quite comprehensive and extensive. Many times a stack of paper eight to 10 inches thick is required in order to capture all of the physiologic events that occur. If you have a study, ask the technician to show you the recording paper that was used. Because of the amount of information, a considerable effort is needed to review it and to arrive at conclusions. In the past, one to three weeks were required to complete the review of the material generated from one study. Fortunately, many laboratories have been able to change their recording system to a computer based method. The ability to record the data from the study on a computer allows for a rapid analysis and review of the information.

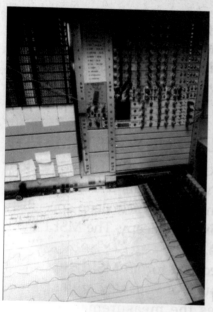

Polysomogram. The physiologic variables of sleep are shown being recorded on paper in this photo. The multiple (poly) sleep (somno) variables recorded (gram) during a night of sleep are called a polysomnogram. These variables may be recorded and saved on a computer instead of paper.

Figure 2-3

If you are scheduled for a polysomnogram, you should be given information advising you of the location of the laboratory, the time of the study, and what preparations, if any, to make.

A sleep study usually will consist of one of two possible patterns. One pattern is sleeping a full night uninterrupted in the laboratory. Usually after a full night of sleep, the following day is observed in the laboratory with a series of naps. The naps form another test called a Multiple Sleep Latency Test or MSLT.

A second pattern that a sleep test often takes occurs when significant sleep apnea is present. If a person has very significant sleep apnea, it will be apparent after a few hours of sleep. In those situations, they would be awakened during the night and a form of treatment called nasal CPAP (pronounced See PAP) would be started (see page 94).

Many patients need more than one night in the sleep laboratory. A second and rarely a third night of study may be required. If your condition is diagnosed as a significant sleep disorder, follow-up studies of your sleep may be required in the future.

MULTIPLE SLEEP LATENCY TEST (MSLT)

The Multiple Sleep Latency Test (MSLT) is another tool for physicians who work with patients with sleep disorders. A frequent complaint with which sleep specialists deal is the problem of being too sleepy. The MSLT measures excessive sleepiness.

If you have been scheduled for an MSLT study, you will be asked to spend much of your day at the laboratory. The study involves the measurement of your tendency to fall asleep several times during a day. Commonly, an MSLT will be performed the day following the night a polysomnogram was performed. Electrodes for the measurement of the EEG will be attached to your head in order to measure your brain waves. If the MSLT follows a polysomnogram, the electrodes from the night study will be left in place. The MSLT study will be carried out several times during the day. You will lie in a quiet room and be asked to sleep while adjustments and measurements are made. Later, you will be awakened and asked to leave the laboratory for a time, only to return

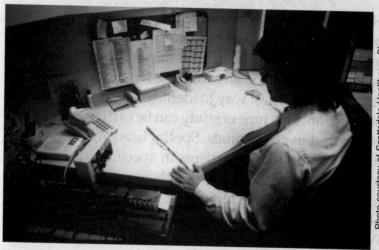

Photo courtesy of Scottsdale Healthcare Shea

Analyzing the Study. Analysis of the sleep study requires a technician to look at each 30 second period of sleep (960 periods for an 8 hour study). The technician notes the stage of sleep, the cardiac status, the respiratory status, and oxygen level for each of these periods. The information is summarized for the study's final report. This photo shows a study being analyzed. Figure 2-4

later for a repeat period of testing. A typical MSLT study will include four such periods of observation during the day.

The sleep physician gains information into your sleepiness by analyzing these periods of observation.

MISCELLANEOUS PROCEDURES

There are a number of other procedures that may be required in evaluating someone with sleep disorders. These include blood testing, lung function testing, laryngoscopy, and radiographic views of the head and neck.

Lung Function Testing (Pulmonary Function Tests) are often needed. A major cause of sleep problems is obstruction of the airway during sleep. It is called sleep apnea. In most cases, the obstruction is not present while awake.

However, there may be mechanical causes of this type of problem including enlarged tonsils, adenoids or abnormal growths in the throat. After the physical exam, if there is concern about the airway, lung function testing is the simplest and easiest way to identify a mechanical airway obstruction. This type of study can be carried out in many offices and in all hospitals. Special head and neck x-rays may be requested for patients in specific circumstances. In individuals with sleep apnea, there are a variety of techniques that have been reported to be useful for evaluation of possible mechanical obstruction in the upper airway. While these studies are not used routinely, selected patients may be chosen for special radiographic views of the head and neck.

Laryngoscopy is a test in which a physician views the upper airway with an instrument that allows evaluation of obstruction in these airways. It can be done in physicians' offices, outpatient facilities, or hospitals. Most often, it is done with local anesthesia and mild sedation. Anesthetic is placed in the nose and mouth. After anesthesia has been achieved, a viewing scope is placed through the nose or mouth into the pharynx. From this area, the entire throat, back portion of the nose, and the larynx can be viewed.

The Evaluation of Sleep Problems
CHAPTER SUMMARY

CHECK YOURSELF
➤ Educate yourself
  —Read about sleep disorders
  —Talk to family and friends
➤ Take a self test
  —Epworth Sleepiness Scale
  —Keep a diary of your sleep
➤ Record your sleep
  —Tape-record the sounds of your sleep
  —Videotape your sleep

DO YOU HAVE A PROBLEM?
➤ Change any bad sleep habits
➤ See a professional for advice

WORKING WITH YOUR PHYSICIAN
➤ Have a list of your medications.
➤ Complete a diary of your sleep before your visit.
➤ Be ready to answer questions regarding sleep, naps, caffeine, alcohol, meals and exercise.
➤ Have your mate attend with you.

TESTING FOR SLEEP PROBLEMS
➤ Sleep study (polysomnography)
  —An all night observation of sleep
  —May be interrupted for a trial of nasal constant positive airway pressure.
➤ Multiple Sleep Latency Testing (MSLT)
  —A series of daytime naps in the laboratory
  —Usually done after a sleep study
➤ Other tests might be needed

TYPES OF
SLEEP PROBLEMS

If you think you or a loved one has a sleep disorder, you can find out and learn more about the problem. Most sleep disorders are easily understood because the types of problems are classified by the symptoms they produce. Use this section to identify a sleep disorder and learn about it.

Section II - Types of Sleep Problems

SECTION II

TYPES OF
SLEEP PROBLEMS

If you think you or a loved one has a sleep disorder, you can find out and learn more about the problem. Most sleep disorders are easily understood because types of problems are classified by the symptoms they produce. Use this section to identify a sleep disorder ... learn about it.

...fication of Sleep Disorders

...Sleep (Insomnia)

Chapter Three

Classification of Sleep Disorders

CLASSIFYING SLEEP PROBLEMS

When do you have a sleep problem? The answer is not always obvious. It is reasonable to assume that you may have a problem if you think you do, if the problem persists, and if it affects how you feel during the day.

It is common to have trouble sleeping. Diet, change in work hours, social plans and many other events all rob our sleep. Sometimes it is difficult to separate out simple troubles from a true sleep problem. Occasionally, those simple troubles with sleep — caused by conflicts with family or social demands — become such a part of our lives that more permanent sleep problems develop. There are serious medical sleep problems that can affect our health and our length of life. If you are concerned, seek help from a professional.

Separating sleep problems into a classification system helps to understand them, and there are several ways to do this. The most practical and widely-used is based upon a person's complaints. For someone with a sleep problem, a system based upon complaints is helpful. Learning more about the conditions which may produce the symptoms will help you decide what steps to take next and when professional help can be of assistance.

The classification of sleep disorders based on symptoms includes four groups. Simply stated, a person can complain of sleeping too little, sleeping too much, sleeping at the wrong time or doing unusual things during sleep. It is important to note that a specific type of sleep disorder, for example, sleep apnea syndrome, can produce different symptoms in different individuals.

How do your complaints fit into the classification system? Once you have a good idea what type of problems you are experiencing, then a review of that group can suggest some possible reasons for your problem. For example, if you have a problem going to sleep, staying asleep or getting enough sleep at night, then you should review the next chapter — Too Little Sleep (Insomnia) — for a listing of the frequent causes of those symptoms. On the other hand, if sleeping too long, falling asleep when you want to be awake, being sleepy all day or having attacks of sleep best describes your symptoms, then chapter five will list the types of problems that commonly produce those complaints.

The last two categories of sleep-related symptoms are often the most dramatic. Sleeping at the wrong time includes people who spend their hours of sleep at times other than expected or wanted. They will sleep their eight hours in the morning, in the afternoon or the early evening, but they will be awake and fine the remaining sixteen hours of their awake time. An interesting group of disorders can cause these situations as you will see in chapter six. The most common problem, jet lag, is covered further in chapter fifteen.

Unusual actions while asleep occur more often than might be expected. The acts include ones as simple as talking or as complex as walking through the house. Rarely does violent activity occur. If your sleep problems include activities during sleep, start by reviewing chapter seven.

Our discussion of sleep problems will follow the outline of this classification system. Each group of disorders along with the problems from that group will be briefly reviewed. In later chapters, the most common sleep disorders will be presented in more detail.

Classification of Sleep Disorders
CHAPTER SUMMARY

SLEEPING TOO LITTLE

➤ Major complaint - Difficulty going to sleep

➤ Typical problem - Insomnia

SLEEPING TOO MUCH

➤ Major complaint - Falling asleep during the day

➤ Typical problem - Sleep Apnea

SLEEPING AT THE WRONG TIME

➤ Major complaint - Needing to sleep at wrong or inappropriate times

➤ Typical problem - Jet lag

DOING UNUSUAL THINGS WHILE ASLEEP

➤ Major complaint - Doing things while asleep

➤ Typical problem - Sleepwalking

Chapter Four

Too Little Sleep (Insomnia)

TOO LITTLE SLEEP

All of us suffer from too little sleep many times throughout our lives. Social events, illnesses and anxieties all interrupt our sleep. It has been estimated that during any year, one-third of the population suffers from significant problems going to sleep or staying asleep for some period of time. While the cause of most of these episodes is clear to us and the episodes end on their own, sometimes the causes are not clear and the problem persists.

Difficulty going to sleep, staying asleep, and going back to sleep are all grouped together. Problems with going to sleep occur when the time we choose to go to bed does not match our ability to go to sleep. Sometimes people go to bed and wait for sleep while at other times they just wait to go to bed when they feel sleepy. Social and work schedules may require an early start to their day. Others are able to go to sleep when they want to go to bed; however, they may awake during the night for unclear reasons and be unable to return to sleep. Repeated awakenings may be part of the problem.

These problems may be caused by many conditions. The common term used to describe these symptoms is insomnia. However, when used by medical personnel the technical definition of insomnia is more complex.

The purpose of this chapter is to list and describe the major causes of insomnia symptoms. Many of these problems are described in more detail in Section III. A general description of some causes follows.

Psychophysiologic

The problems of psychophysiologic insomnia can be separated into those of short duration and those which are long-term disorders. These are the most common reasons for sleeping difficulties.

Problems of short duration are frequent and well-known. Examples include difficulty sleeping because of anxiety brought on by family, work or social situations. A death in the family, change in jobs, or an argument with a friend can all affect the ability to sleep.

Problems are considered long-term when they last longer than three months. These problems usually cannot be related to specific events and no medical causes for the sleeping problem can be found. These individuals are commonly described as having chronic insomnia. This topic is covered in more detail in chapter twelve.

Drugs - Caffeine, Alcohol, Medications, and others

Many drugs or chemicals may affect our sleep. Often, they are a part of our everyday life. The most common are caffeine and alcohol. Caffeine delays sleep and prevents restful sleep. Alcohol brings on sleep but prevents restful sleep and may cause early awakening with difficulty going back to sleep. Many medications have effects on the quality of sleep. Both over the counter medications and prescription medications can result in poor sleep. Illicit drug use commonly produces problems with sleep both during usage and in the withdrawal period. The effects of drug habits on sleep are covered in more detail in chapter eleven.

Medical Illnesses and Disorders

When ill, one may find it difficult to sleep. Many types of medical illnesses interfere with sleep. The pain of arthritis or an injury, nasal congestion from the common cold or allergies, and coughing from bronchitis are all common reasons for a poor night's sleep. Chronic illnesses frequently produce sleeping problems. For example, sleep is affected by shortness of breath associated with heart failure, asthma and emphysema; nausea from abdominal problems, or discomfort from cancer or back pain all interfere with sleep. Many medications used to treat these same chronic conditions may further disturb sleep.

Environmental

Problems in the environment produce difficulty sleeping. These are usually apparent and sleep improves when the environmental problem is corrected. Examples might include living next to a train track, sleeping with the lights or television on, or using a worn-out mattress. Sometimes habits adopted over a period of time have an adverse effect on sleep. Watching television in bed can start as a way to pass a few minutes prior to sleep and progress over a few years to keeping someone from sleeping well.

The role of behavior and habits on sleep is reviewed in chapter eleven.

Perception

Some individuals who feel they are having inadequate sleep, actually sleep normally. When tested, their sleep, including length of time asleep, the sleep stages, and number of awakenings is normal. These individuals often overestimate the time it takes to go to sleep, the number of times they awaken during the night, and the length of time they are awake while trying to sleep. They underestimate the amount of time they actually sleep. It is important to be evaluated thoroughly by a physician familiar with sleep problems to exclude other medical reasons for the sleep complaints.

Psychiatric

Individuals with psychiatric disorders frequently have problems sleeping. Examples include schizophrenia, mania, and depression, that when treated often lead to improved sleep. Even mild forms of anxiety and depression that do not require treatment with medications may affect sleep.

Periodic Limb Movements

Rhythmic shaking of the muscles in the legs and arms may occur during sleep. These muscle contractions vary in strength. Sometimes they are strong enough to disturb sleep and even wake the sleeper. Furthermore, limb movements may be strong enough to disturb another sleeper in the same bed. Medications are available that help to control the movements. Chapter fourteen has more on this subject.

Sleep Apnea

This breathing disorder is a very common problem during sleep and has serious medical and health consequences. For short periods while asleep, the breathing stops (apnea) and the quality of rest is affected. The individual may feel like he is sleeping too little as a result. However, most individuals with sleep apnea complain of sleeping too much. This disorder affects a significant portion of the population and is a major public health problem. One section of this book is dedicated to cover the subject (chapters nine and ten).

Restless Legs

Sufferers from this condition experience restlessness of their legs as they try to go to sleep. The feeling may be one of irritation, tingling, or just the need to move the legs. The sensations seem to be relieved by movement and changing the position of the legs. Those who suffer from restless legs have difficulty becoming comfortable enough to fall asleep easily. The common types of leg and arm problems that affect sleep are reviewed in more detail in chapter fourteen.

Too Little Sleep
CHAPTER SUMMARY

Insomnia — The symptoms of trouble going to sleep, staying asleep, or going back to sleep.

Causes of Insomnia

➤ Psychophysiologic — Problems resulting from worry, anxiety, stress or unknown reasons

➤ Drugs — Caffeine, Alcohol, Medications and Illicit drugs

➤ Medical Illnesses — A frequent cause

➤ Environmental — Noise, light and temperature

➤ Perception — Sleeping more than they realize

➤ Psychiatric — Mental illnesses and the drugs used to treat them

➤ Periodic Limb Movements — Rhythmic jerks of limbs which disturb sleep

➤ Sleep Apnea Syndrome — Repeated breathing problems during sleep

➤ Restless legs — Irritation of the legs which causes frequent movements and position changes

Chapter Five

Excessive Sleepiness

SLEEPING TOO MUCH

A common problem is sleeping more than necessary — sleeping too much. This symptom occurs more frequently than you might expect. Often, someone's need for more sleep will not be obvious to others. Sleepiness can be temporarily suppressed and put off until a later time. It may only occur with certain events or activities. Surprisingly, the symptoms may not even be recognized by the person who has them. When sleepiness increases slowly over months or years, the person may not recognize they are sleeping too much. Family and friends are the ones who bring it to their attention. Just as surprising, sometimes the problems with sleepiness are so severe that the person cannot stay awake to describe them, but in fact falls asleep in the act of explaining them.

As with all symptoms, a number of reasons for excessive sleepiness exist. This chapter reviews the common causes. Many of the conditions are similar to the ones that produce symptoms of sleeping too little. Remember that many identical conditions affect people differently. One person with a problem might feel that he is sleeping too much while another will feel that he is not sleeping enough.

Sleep-disordered Breathing

These disorders were described (discovered) by modern medicine in the 1960s. However, they have been with us throughout human history. Sleep apnea is the major breathing problem during sleep and represents a serious health problem.

During sleep, breathing can be temporarily obstructed. The obstructions can completely stop the breathing (apnea) or partially obstruct it (hypopnea). These events disturb the quality and quantity of sleep, produce low oxygen levels, cause mental deterioration, and worsen high blood pressure. The condition that results from a large number of these events — sleep apnea syndrome — is diagnosable and treatable. After treatment, improvement is often dramatic.

Sometimes an apnea occurs simply because breathing just stops and there is no obstruction to the airway. This type of apnea is called a central apnea. It occurs because the brain forgets to tell the chest to breathe. These serious disorders are the subject of section III of this book (chapters nine and ten).

Narcolepsy

Narcolepsy is a disease of the brain with a strong genetic influence that involves the brain's control over wakefulness and sleepiness. This disease is characterized by sleep attacks. A sleep attack is a sudden onset of sleep or the irresistible need for sleep. The episodes may be associated with muscle weakness and sometimes result in complete or partial physical collapse. These episodes are called cataplexy. They can be brought on by strong emotions or stress. Some individuals with narcolepsy have daytime sleepiness in addition to their sleep attacks. Further information can be found in chapter thirteen.

Drugs — Medications, Alcohol and Others

Many medications can make you sleepy. Antihistamines are a common example. If you are overly sleepy and taking medications, review your drugs carefully with your physician. A simple change in medications may improve your alertness. Alcohol affects alertness and brings on sleep, although sleep after alcohol can be fitful and disturbed. Illicit drugs may bring on excessive sleep in addition to many other problems. Chapter eleven reviews the effects of drugs on sleep.

Medical Illnesses

Many illnesses and medical disorders may be associated with sleepiness. Diseases as serious as brain tumors or as troublesome as hay fever may result in an increased need for sleep. Following the flu, bronchitis, or pneumonia, more sleep may be needed for a period of time. Another example is low thyroid activity (hypothyroidism). Individuals whose thyroid glands do not produce enough hormones can suffer many changes including an increase in their need for sleep.

Psychiatric Disorders

Individuals with psychiatric problems can have excessive sleepiness as a result of their diseases. Examples include depression and schizophrenia. These situations represent difficult problems since the medications used to treat these diseases may produce some of the same sleep symptoms.

Perceptions

Judgement of our own sleep quality may be incorrect. Sometimes, a physician's careful review of personal sleep habits (the duration, time of day and changes in sleep over days) and medical evaluation fails to reveal any excessive sleepiness. Although one may feel that he sleeps too much and is excessively sleepy, no evidence can be found to indicate any abnormality. In such situations, it is important that an experienced physician reviews the symptoms and evaluates for other possible explanations.

Periodic Limb Movements

This disorder, rhythmic shaking of the limb muscles (usually legs) may cause difficulty going to sleep. In addition, the shaking may occur during sleep and disturb the quality of the sleep. If a night of sleep is disturbed by a large number of limb movements, excessive sleepiness during the day may result. Chapter fourteen covers this subject in more detail.

Naturally Long Sleeper

The amount of sleep needed to restore and refresh is different for each of us. If someone has a need for more sleep than they think is normal, it can cause worry. A consistent requirement for a sleep time of nine to ten hours occurs in some normal people. A long sleep time needed to feel refreshed in the morning is not a disease nor should it be considered a problem. Consult your physician to confirm any questions or suspicions you might have.

Idiopathic Hypersomnolence

There are some individuals who have serious problems sleeping too much and the cause cannot be found. When no specific cause for their excessive sleepiness can be found, the process is called idiopathic hypersomnolence. People with the problem often sleep both at night and during the day. They fall asleep at dinner, during a conversation or in front of the television. The sleepiness is present much of the day and at inappropriate times. This problem needs careful evaluation by a physician experienced in sleep disorders.

Sleeping Too Much
CHAPTER SUMMARY

Sleeping too much — Falling asleep at the wrong time or too early or staying asleep for too long.

Causes

➤ Sleep Apnea
  —Breathing temporarily obstructed
  —Causes interrupted sleep
  —Produces low oxygen levels, heart and memory problems

➤ Narcolepsy
  —Sudden onset of sleep
  —Irresistible need for sleep
  —Episodes of weakness

➤ Drugs (medications, alcohol) — Many

➤ Medical Illnesses — Serious or minor illness

➤ Psychiatric Disorders — Both the disorders and their treatments

➤ Perception — Sleeping less than realized

➤ Periodic Limb Movements — Uncontrollable jerking of the limbs interrupting sleep

➤ Naturally Long Sleeper — Requires more time for sleep

➤ Idiopathic Hypersomnolence — Excessive sleepiness of unknown cause

Chapter Six

Sleeping at the Wrong Time

SLEEPING AT THE WRONG TIME

This interesting group of disorders includes problems with the time of day when we sleep. Two factors seem to control our need for sleep. The first is our circadian rhythm, the biological time clock that controls our body's functions. It tells us when to sleep and usually runs on a 24-hour schedule. The second can be called the "exhaustion effect." The amount of activity performed and the amount of previous sleep work together to determine this effect. The combination of these factors causes us to sleep. Usually the average person sleeps once every twenty-four hours for a period of approximately eight hours during the night. Chapter one reviews the variations of normal sleep. There are situations and problems when sleep occurs at the wrong time.

The disorders in this group represent situations where the controlling factors do not result in normal sleep times. Sleep does occur and may be of normal duration and pattern, but it occurs at the wrong time of day. The symptom of sleeping at the wrong time or needing to sleep at the wrong time can be due to simple or complex problems. Rapid travel to a new time zone results in sleep problems. Problems can develop because the circadian cycle is abnormal in length or the sleep cycle has become set at the wrong time.

Jet Lag

Modern travel moves us rapidly over long distances. Leaving home today at noon, you could be halfway around the world in 24 hours. But, if you are there in 24 hours, the local time will be midnight, not noon. Your body's clock — its circadian clock — will think it is noon, but it will be midnight locally. Your body will want to be awake, but it is time to sleep.

In the new location, you feel alert at night and sleepy during the day. You have jet lag, and it will take time to readjust your internal clock. Jet lag is a self-correcting problem that can be minimized by planning. For some tips and further information see chapter fifteen.

Shift Work

A problem similar to jet lag happens to workers who shift their work times. If you work the day shift for some time, but are temporarily shifted to the night shift, your body's clock will need time to adjust. The first night on the night shift, your body's clock will say it is time to sleep when you need to be working. If you are not prepared, the need for sleep may be hard to resist. When working nights or at times normal for sleep, time for sleep must be allowed during the daytime. Working the late night shift should be done for an extended period to allow the body's circadian rhythm to readjust. Changing the hours worked can cause some significant sleeping problems.

Abnormal Circadian Rhythms

Some individuals have biological clocks which do not run on a 24-hour schedule. Their circadian clock may run on a longer or shorter schedule. For example, the circadian clock may run at a 26-hour schedule. The clock would tell your body that you should sleep every 26 hours.

If your 26-hour biological clock has you sleeping well tonight, then you will not want to sleep again for another 26 hours — two hours later each day. Each night you would want to go to sleep two hours later. After six days, the time of day that your circadian rhythm tells you to sleep is the middle of the day.

The circadian rhythm may be slow as in the above example, it may be fast, or it may be totally disorganized. Complete disorganization is seen as a characteristic of the young infant and in those who suffer from Alzheimer's disease.

Delayed Sleep Phase Syndrome

In this situation, sleep begins late in the night and lasts into the daylight hours. Sleep might begin at three or four in the morning and last until noon the next day. Sleep, when measured in the sleep laboratory, is normal, just the time of day when it occurs is inappropriate. The person feels refreshed upon awaking, however, when they try to awake at an earlier time to go work or for other activities, the need for sleep is almost impossible to overcome. Attempts at sleeping nighttime hours fail. The person is often sleepy during the day when forced to live an eight to five day. The situation may develop out of environmental or social demands, but the circadian rhythm becomes abnormal and probably makes readjustment difficult.

Advanced Sleep Phase Syndrome

This is an unusual problem in that sleep begins earlier than desired. The person falls asleep early, typically, before they want to go to sleep. The sleep is normal and of adequate length. While sleep results in feeling refreshed upon awaking, morning comes at a very early hour of the day. Typically, the person is unable to stay awake in the evening even when necessary, but is very awake and ready for activity at an early hour — three or four in the morning.

Sleeping at the Wrong Time
CHAPTER SUMMARY

JET LAG
➤ Occurs when traveling through time zones
➤ Biological clock conflicts with time of day
➤ Temporary — corrects in a few days

SHIFT WORK
➤ Caused by changing work schedule
➤ Biological clock conflicts with work time
➤ Temporary — corrects with time

ABNORMAL CIRCADIAN RHYTHM
➤ Biological clock not on a 24 hour cycle
➤ Desire to sleep varies
    —Circadian rhythm in control
    —Time of day not important

DELAYED SLEEP PHASE SYNDROME
➤ Normal sleep and sleep duration
➤ Sleep occurs at late night to midday
➤ Cause unclear

ADVANCED SLEEP PHASE SYNDROME
➤ Normal sleep and sleep duration
➤ Sleep onset occurs early and ends early
➤ Cause unclear

Chapter Seven

Unusual Movements During Sleep

The Parasomnias

When sleep problems are discussed, the disorders in this group are always subjects of major interest. Some of these disorders have such dramatic presentations that we cannot help but be interested in their nature. They vary from the simple and curious to the frightening and dangerous. They are most often observed by others, but the sufferer may be aware of some of the events and activities. Medically, there are similarities in the manner in which these disorders are thought to occur. The brain is thought to lose some control over the sleep process during certain stages of sleep or when changing from one stage to another. The body will carry out certain physical acts during sleep that are not part of normal sleep.

Sleepwalking

The person who gets up and walks during sleep is a typical example of these disorders. The behavior appears controlled but has no active purpose. Normal muscle activities occur. Usually, the patients do not injure themselves, but they can fall, run into furniture, bump their heads or have other minor injuries.

The episodes last a variable period of time but commonly, just a few minutes, usually during the first third of the night. The person may wander for a short period or he may rush around. He may dress, open doors, or perform simple repetitive acts. He may seem to be awake when observed. The person is hard to arouse during the activity and will not remember the event in the morning. After these activities, the person may return to bed, lie down on the floor or somewhere else and then return to normal sleep.

Sleepwalking occurs almost exclusively in the pediatric age range. It is commonly associated with sleep terrors.

Sleep Terrors

Sleep terrors are events that when seen, suggest the person is having a severely frightening event while sleeping. During sleep, the individual will suddenly start shouting out or performing some activity of a violent or threatening nature. The activity can be kicking, beating with the fists, jumping out of bed, running into walls, or screaming out. These activities frequently result in injury to the individual or bedmate. The terror ends as rapidly as it begins with the person returning to sleep. In the morning or upon awaking, there is no memory of the event, but an occasional sense of dread remains.

Sleep terrors are more common in children than in adults. In children, the attacks may be brought on by fatigue, illness or stress, however, most have no clear cause. In adults, psychological problems such as chronic anxiety are more frequently seen. In any age group, adequate sleep and avoidance of fatigue seem to be helpful.

Sleep Talking

Talking during sleep occurs commonly and represents one form of these disorders. Most often just a word or phrase that seems to have no meaning is spoken. It may be slurred, garbled or unclear. Contrary to popular belief, secrets or important information is not poured out. Most sleep talk makes no sense to those who hear it. Sleep talking may occur with sleep walking or sleep terrors, but occurs most frequently as an isolated benign occurrence.

Rhythmic Movement Disorder

This interesting disorder occurs in children and consists of repeated unusual movements at the onset of sleep but disappears within a short time after sleep begins. Headbanging against the bed or mattress, rocking of the body repetitively back and forth, and rolling of the head or legs are all types of movements that have been described. The disorder resolves with time and treatment other than protection from injury is usually not needed.

Confusional Arousals

There are individuals who have recurrent problems with confusion when awaking. They will not know where they are or what time of day it is upon awaking. Speech often will be slurred and thinking will be slowed. The situation is most commonly seen in children and resolves after puberty. Children who have sleep terrors or sleep-walking commonly also have confusional arousals. Rarely, it can occur in adults, usually when they suffer from sleep apnea syndrome.

REM Behavior Disorders

This problem has features of sleepwalking and sleep terrors. However, it is primarily seen in older individuals. They may appear to wake during sleep and seem to be acting out dreams. Activities such as shoveling, fighting or other behaviors may be acted out. Often the behavior is of a violent nature and the individuals may injure themselves. The problem differs from those described above in that the patients are older and may have evidence of a brain disorder. Furthermore, REM is the stage of sleep during which these events occur.

Unusual Movements During Sleep
CHAPTER SUMMARY

This group of disorders, called parasomnias, is thought to be related to problems with changing stages of sleep and the control of muscular activity.

SLEEPWALKING
➤ Usually a problem of children
➤ Movement around room or house while asleep
➤ No memory of events the next morning

(continued on next page)

Unusual Movements During Sleep
CHAPTER SUMMARY *(continued)*

SLEEP TERRORS
➤ Waking with shouting, screaming or violent behavior
➤ May result in injury to the person
➤ Most common in children

SLEEP TALKING
➤ Most common form of parasomnias
➤ Speech often slurred or garbled
➤ Usually makes no sense when heard

RHYTHMIC MOVEMENT DISORDER
➤ A problem of childhood
➤ Repetitive movements at the onset of sleep such as head banging, body rocking and body rolling
➤ May be associated with sleep terrors and sleep-walking

CONFUSIONAL AROUSALS
➤ Confusion on awaking
➤ Usually a childhood disorder
➤ May be seen with sleep apnea syndrome

REM BEHAVIOR DISORDERS
➤ Occurs in older adults
➤ Seem to be acting out dreams
➤ Often violent behavior

SLEEP APNEA SYNDROME

Sleep apnea is a major sleep disorder with serious health consequences. This entire section covers the problem of sleep apnea, its diagnosis and treatment.

Chapter Eight

Sleep Apnea—
What Is It?

INTRODUCTION TO SLEEP APNEA

During sleep, our bodily functions continue. Our hearts beat, we breathe, and our kidneys fill our bladders. Breathing problems during sleep are a major cause of sleep-related complaints.

Sleep apnea was described as a medical problem only 40 years ago, although described in literature for over a thousand years. It is the most common reason for excessive sleepiness. Sleep apnea is the disease that sleep specialists deal with most often.

After sleep apnea was discovered, other forms of breathing problems during sleep were recognized. These problems may cause symptoms just like those of sleep apnea. The breathing disorders during sleep are related and are similar. *Sleep apnea* is the term applied when breathing stops for short periods while asleep. *Sleep hypopnea* is the term applied when breathing is significantly reduced (but does not stop) for short periods while asleep. *Upper airway resistance* is the term applied when breathing difficulties (labored but not stopped nor significantly reduced) caused by problems in the mouth, throat or nose result in partially waking up from sleep.

Each of these problems can affect us in two ways. Interrupting our sleep is the first. If our breathing is affected often enough, we may not get enough good sleep. Although we sleep in bed a long time, it may not be enough of the right kind of sleep. You can spend eight to ten hours asleep, but without the right kind of sleep, you will still be sleepy when you awake. Normal sleep consists of sleep in several different levels or stages. Breathing problems during sleep may prevent you from getting enough of the deep stages of sleep. Lack of deep sleep at night will cause sleepiness and tiredness during the day.

Breathing problems during sleep can cause arousals. When asleep, if breathing problems develop, you can wake up partially. You may not wake up enough that you are aware of being awake. This is called an arousal. When arousals occur, your sleep becomes lighter. When measured, the sleep stages change from deeper sleep to lighter sleep. You have aroused in your sleep. If you are aroused often enough, your sleep is not restful and you are still tired in the morning.

The second major way breathing problems affect us during sleep is by causing low oxygen levels in the blood. Low oxygen levels during the night can have several different effects on how we feel and on our health.

Low oxygen levels will be sensed by the body and breathing will be stimulated. We breathe harder and stronger when oxygen levels are low. Repeated low oxygen levels can cause problems with memory, thinking and concentration.

Low oxygen levels can cause the blood pressure in the arteries that take blood to the lungs (the pulmonary arteries) to be high. If the oxygen level stays low enough for a long enough period of time, permanent changes can develop in the pulmonary arteries that result in heart failure.

Sleep Apnea Syndrome is the name of the disease caused by breathing irregularities during sleep. Apneas, hypopneas, or upper airway resistance, alone or in combination, may produce the disease. To understand more about breathing problems during sleep, we first need to learn a little of our anatomy and how we breathe.

BREATHING PROBLEMS DURING SLEEP

They are common problems.
They are caused by complete or partial obstruction to breathing during sleep.
They affect a person by:
  —Interrupting sleep
  —Lowering blood oxygen levels.
The disease caused by these events is called the *Sleep Apnea Syndrome.*

ANATOMY AND PHYSIOLOGY OF SLEEP APNEA

To understand sleep apnea and its causes, it is helpful to know how we breathe and which parts of our bodies are used in breathing.

Breathing

Breathing occurs regularly every minute, every day of our lives, while we are asleep as well as during our waking hours.

Breathing performs two functions for our bodies. It serves to get oxygen into the body and carry carbon dioxide out.

Air enters our body through the nose or mouth, enters the throat, passes through the voice box, enters the trachea and bronchi, and ends its journey in the lungs. There, oxygen enters the blood and carbon dioxide leaves the blood and enters the air to be exhaled.

Breathing takes effort. To get air into the lungs requires work. The work is done by the muscles of the diaphragm and chest wall. The muscles expand the chest and air is sucked into the lungs.

Exhalation is easier. No work is required. We exhale by relaxing the same respiratory muscles. Air passes out of the lungs as the chest returns to a resting position.

In and out. We breathe eight to twelve breaths per minute our entire lives. Our breathing is regulated, coordinated, and adjusted by our brain. Breathing is automatic. If we need to breathe more or less, the brain acts as a regulator.

Anatomy of Respiration

To understand breathing disorders, it is important to know about the parts of the body involved. The respiratory system is connected to the outside air by both the nose and mouth. They connect to the throat which is connected to the voice box, windpipe and lungs.

The *nasal passage* and the mouth meet in the *throat*. They are separated by the *palate*. In the front it contains bone and is called the *hard palate*. In the back, the palate is soft and movable. This part of the palate is called the *soft palate*. A portion of the soft palate extends downward from the palate. It is called the *uvula*.

The *throat* is called the *pharynx* and is divided into three areas. The part where the nose enters the throat is called the *nasopharynx*. The area where the mouth meets the throat is called the *oropharynx*. The part below the oropharynx is called the *hypopharynx*.

At the bottom of the hypopharynx is the *larynx* which contains the *vocal cords* and connects to the *trachea*. The larynx is protected by a flap of tissue called the *epiglottis* which closes during swallowing so that no liquids enter the lungs.

The structures from the nose and mouth to the vocal cords are considered to be the upper airway.

The *tonsils* are located in the upper airway. They are at the entryway to the oropharynx from the mouth and are just below the end of the soft palate.

The lower airway consists of the *trachea*, *bronchi*, and *alveoli*. The *trachea* is the single tube that connects the lungs to the larynx. As the air tubes branch out from the trachea, they are called bronchi. The *bronchi* branch similarly to the limbs on a tree, getting smaller and smaller the further they extend into the lungs. At the end of the bronchi, in the smallest tubes, we find the *alveoli*. The *alveoli* are air sacs which are surrounded by blood vessels. It is in the alveoli that the oxygen is taken up and the carbon dioxide released.

The act of breathing requires work of the chest wall muscles. The *thorax* is a rigid structure surrounded by bones and muscles. The *diaphragm* muscle at the bottom of the thorax serves as a pump. When it contracts, it pulls the lungs open and air is drawn into the chest. Muscles between the ribs also help pull air into the lungs. When they contract the thorax expands.

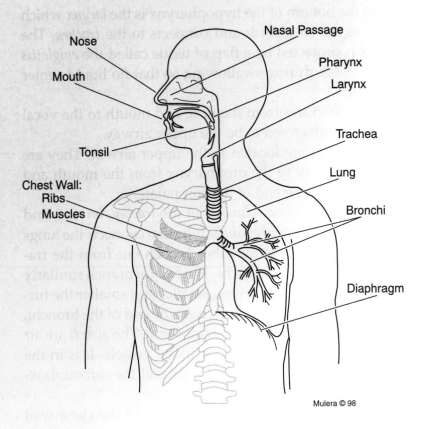

Nasal Passage

Nose

Pharynx

Mouth

Larynx

Trachea

Tonsil

Lung

Chest Wall:
Ribs
Muscles

Bronchi

Diaphragm

Mulera © 98

Respiratory System

Figure 8-1

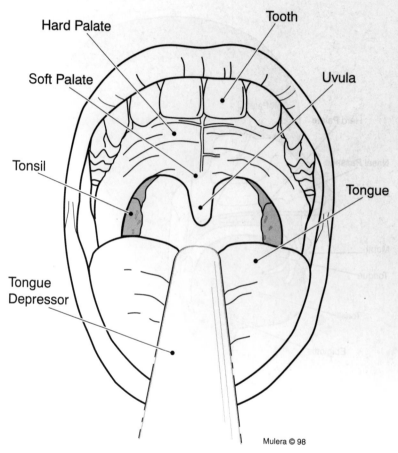

Hard Palate

Tooth

Soft Palate

Uvula

Tonsil

Tongue

Tongue Depressor

Mulera © 98

Mouth and Throat

Figure 8-2

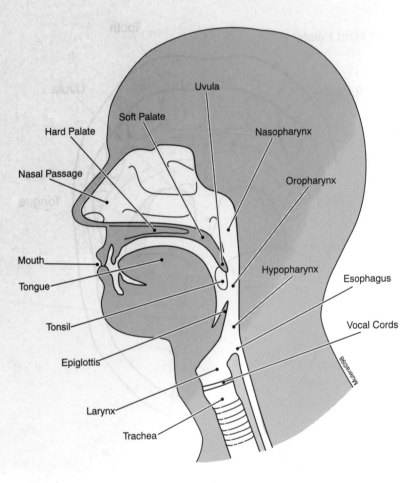

Upper Airway

Figure 8-3

BREATHING PROBLEMS DURING SLEEP

Breathing during sleep is identical to breathing while awake. The respiratory muscles contract (we inhale) and air moves into the lungs. We relax and the air leaves the lungs (we exhale). Changes in breathing while we sleep include obstructive sleep apnea, central sleep apnea, sleep hypopnea, and upper airway resistance.

Obstructive Sleep Apnea Events

Breathing is interrupted when apnea is present. Apnea is defined as the absence of breathing for ten seconds. The most common type of apnea is obstructive apnea.

Obstructive apnea usually occurs when the upper airway closes. The act of breathing continues. The chest wall and diaphragm move, but no air goes into the lungs. Obstructive apneas occur as sleep enters the deeper levels. The deep sleep causes the muscles in the throat to relax excessively and the airway in the pharynx closes.

When the airway obstructs and apnea occurs, it takes a few seconds for the body to sense that it is not breathing normally. Once the body senses it is not getting enough oxygen and eliminating enough carbon dioxide, the breathing efforts increase. The stronger efforts at breathing overcome the obstruction and air starts to move into the lungs again. The sleep levels change as the obstruction is overcome. Sleep becomes lighter and the effort to breathe may cause the person to awaken.

Snoring is a common sign of obstructive sleep apnea. A change in the loudness of the snoring occurs as apnea occurs. The snoring will gradually become softer and softer. When apnea occurs, snoring will disappear. When the increased effort of breathing overcomes the obstruction, snoring will start again with a loud snort. This change in snoring is one of the most important signs of sleep apnea.

Obstructive Sleep Hypopnea Events

A decrease in the breathing is termed hypopnea. Breathing becomes more shallow but does not totally stop as it does with apnea.

The mechanism of hypopnea is the same as that causing obstructive apnea. The difference is that complete obstruction does not occur. Breathing is reduced but not stopped.

Most people with breathing problems during sleep have both apneas and hypopneas.

Upper Airway Resistance Events

Upper airway resistance events are like sleep apnea and sleep hypopnea and may cause a similar illness.

Upper airway resistance episodes are mild obstructive events. These episodes are so mild that hypopnea or apnea does not occur.

These events cause disturbances in sleep which can result in some of the same symptoms and problems that trouble patients with sleep apnea and sleep hypopnea.

Central Sleep Apnea Events

Central sleep apneas account for a very small percent of sleep apnea episodes. No obstruction occurs with central sleep apnea. When central apnea occurs, the breathing just stops. The brain forgets to tell the chest muscles to breathe, so that no air is pulled into the lungs.

Central sleep apnea events may be seen in normal people and those with obstructive sleep apnea syndrome. Rarely, the events occur often enough during the night to cause symptoms and problems on their own.

NORMAL SLEEP

This graph shows events which occur over three minutes of sleep. The breathing movements of the chest are recorded as chest wall movements. The air flow represents air entering and leaving the nose and mouth. The oxygen level is recorded continuously. When snoring occurs it is marked on the next line. The depth of sleep is indicated along the bottom line.

During sleep the chest moves methodically. As a result, air moves in and out of the lungs in a regular pattern. The blood oxygen level remains relatively constant with only an occasional change and remains within normal limits. No snoring is recorded. The depth of sleep changes only occasionally.

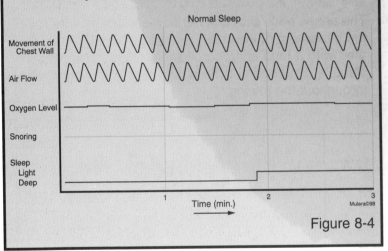

Normal Sleep

Figure 8-4

OBSTRUCTIVE SLEEP APNEA

This graph shows events which occur over three minutes during sleep. The breathing movements of the chest are recorded as chest wall movements. The air flow represents air entering and leaving the nose and mouth. The oxygen level is recorded continuously. When snoring occurs it is marked on the next line. The depth of sleep is indicated along the bottom line.

When obstructive sleep apnea occurs, breathing continues but changes. The chest movements can be seen to increase while the air moving into the lungs decreases and stops. Notice the oxygen levels begin to drop as the air flow decreases. This patient snores loudly, but the snoring decreases and stops as the air entering the lungs decreases and stops also. This period of no air flow is an apnea.

The apnea ends suddenly. Air flow starts suddenly when the movement of the chest is at its greatest. It is associated with a loud snorting or snore sound. The patient's sleep is disturbed and he is aroused. The events recur throughout the tracing.

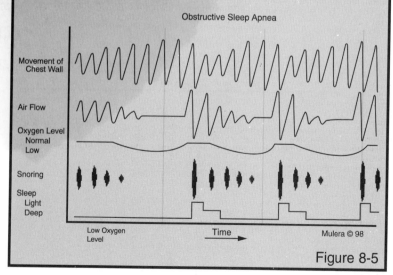

Obstructive Sleep Apnea

Figure 8-5

CENTRAL SLEEP APNEA

This graph shows events which occur over three minutes during sleep. The breathing movements of the chest are recorded as chest wall movements. The air flow represents air entering and leaving the nose and mouth. The oxygen level is recorded continuously. When snoring occurs it is marked on the next line. The depth of sleep is indicated along the bottom line.

When central sleep apnea occurs, breathing stop for short periods of time for unknown reasons. The movements of the chest stop. At the same time air stops moving into the lungs. Slightly later the oxygen level in the blood drops. No snoring is recorded. The depth of sleep changes as a result of these events.

Just as suddenly, the chest begins to move again and the normal findings return. The central apneas are shown to occur four times in the diagram.

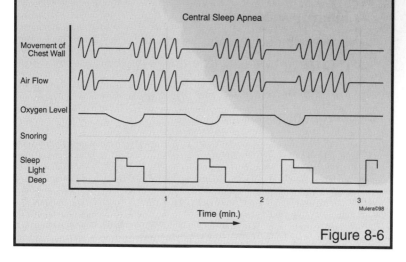

Figure 8-6

Sleep Apnea - What Is It?
CHAPTER SUMMARY

SLEEP APNEA
A breathing problem during sleep

Usually caused by a complete or partial obstruction to breathing during sleep.

- Blockage of the airway in the throat
- Intermittent - lasting a few seconds
- Complete obstruction - apnea
- Partial obstruction - hypopnea

OBSTRUCTIVE SLEEP APNEA SYNDROME
The disease produced when repeated obstructions occur.

- Interrupts sleep
- Lowers blood oxygen levels
- Causes or worsens high blood pressure
- Causes or worsens heart disease
- Frequent accidents

CENTRAL SLEEP APNEA
- An unusual problem where the breathing stops for a few seconds and no obstruction is present.

Chapter Nine

Sleep Apnea Syndrome
— The Disease —

SLEEP APNEA SYNDROME

When apnea or hypopnea events occur often enough during someone's sleep, a medical illness is the result. Sleep apnea syndrome is the term applied to the group of symptoms, signs and findings that people exhibit when they have the illness. It is the disease produced by breathing problems during sleep.

Men have more problems than women. Eight of ten patients with sleep apnea syndrome are males, although the difference lessens as we grow older. Sleep apnea does run in families. Many fathers and sons, and mothers and daughters, share the same problems.

Sleep apnea syndrome is a common condition. It is estimated that up to 10% of the adult population suffer from some degree of sleep apnea syndrome.

Sleep apnea syndrome is usually a disease of the mature or older person. The age at the time of diagnosis is usually greater than 50 years, however, sleep apnea can occur at any age. Younger people with sleep apnea often have it as the result of other medical problems.

SYMPTOMS OF SLEEP APNEA SYNDROME

Someone with sleep apnea syndrome can have a number of symptoms. The most common is sleepiness during the daytime. The complaints vary from fatigue and tiredness to extreme sleepiness. With extreme sleepiness, sleep onset may occur while sitting, talking, working or even eating.

These individuals often fall asleep in the evening after dinner while watching television or reading. After being awakened to go to bed, they fall asleep in bed as soon as they lie down.

Choking can be experienced during sleep. The person awakens suddenly and is unable to breathe. Choking may become so pronounced, that after experiencing it, the person does not return to bed for fear of choking again. People who experience choking often report on their lack of sleep rather than problems with sleeping too much.

Commonly, people with sleep apnea syndrome complain of a poor night's sleep and feeling tired or exhausted in the morning despite an adequate time asleep.

Morning headaches are common. They are thought to be the result of low blood oxygen levels during sleep. The pain is most intense shortly after awakening and clears later in the morning. The pain usually occurs on the top of the head.

People with sleep apnea may complain of confusion in the morning upon awakening, or their spouses notice it in them. When sleep apnea has been present for several years, unexpected problems with memory, concentration and ability to perform mental tasks may be reported.

Since sleep apnea syndrome develops gradually over several years, patients are often able to adjust somewhat to the symptoms. They can change their habits to help cope with the effects. Increasing the amount of caffeine ingested or allowing more time for naps are ways to combat symptoms. As a result, spouses and other family members may be more concerned than the person with the symptoms. It is common for someone with very significant sleep apnea syndrome to have no complaints and think he is just fine.

SIGNS OF SLEEP APNEA SYNDROME

About half the patients with sleep apnea syndrome have a problem with their weight. The extremely obese almost all have sleep apnea syndrome. A neck size of greater than 18 inches is a strong indication of the presence of sleep apnea.

Snoring is a common finding and may be loud or soft. Loud snoring should be considered to be an indication of breathing problems during sleep, but not everyone who snores loudly has sleep apnea. Variation in the snoring is a strong sign of sleep apnea syndrome. Typically the snoring starts with a snort, followed by loud snoring that decreases to soft and then silence, then snort, loud, decreasing to silence, and snort in a repeating pattern.

Hypertension is a common problem among older Americans and it can be caused by sleep apnea syndrome. In patients with other forms of hypertension, sleep apnea syndrome can make the high blood pressure harder to control, can increase blood pressure and can increase the amount of medications required to control the blood pressure.

Many times the spouses or others will report observing apneas. The report of seeing apnea in someone with symptoms of sleep apnea increases the likelihood of the disease being present. Sometimes choking during sleep, thrashing following choking, or snorting are observed. These are strong indications of the presence of sleep-disordered breathing.

SYMPTOMS AND SIGNS OF SLEEP APNEA SYNDROME*

SYMPTOMS

➤ Poor sleep at night

➤ Fatigue or exhaustion in morning

➤ Confusion on awakening

➤ Daytime sleepiness

➤ Choking during sleep

➤ Morning headaches

SIGNS

➤ Obesity

➤ Neck size greater than 18 inches

➤ Snoring

➤ High blood pressure

➤ Apnea or choking during sleep seen by others

*These symptoms and signs suggest the problem of sleep apnea syndrome is present.

CAUSES OF SLEEP APNEA SYNDROME

Sleep apnea syndrome results from repetitive obstruction of the upper airway during sleep. The episodes disturb the quality of sleep and cause low blood oxygen levels. Sleep apnea syndrome can be caused by a number of medical conditions, but most of the time, it occurs alone. When obstructive sleep apnea is the only problem present and no other cause for sleep apnea is found, it is called idiopathic obstructive sleep apnea (obstructive sleep apnea without known cause).

Hypothyroidism

Hypothyroidism, low thyroid hormone levels, is one cause of sleep apnea syndrome. It produces fatigue and exhaustion. Patients who develop sleep apnea problems from low thyroid hormone will have the typical signs and symptoms. Correcting low thyroid levels to normal will cause sleep apnea to disappear.

Physical Upper Airway Obstruction

Obstruction in the upper airway can cause sleep apnea. There are several ways that obstruction can occur. The most common is from enlarged tonsils.

The tonsils can increase to several times normal size. They are located in the oropharynx at the important junction with the nasopharynx. Large tonsils may cause no problems when a person is in the upright position or when awake and lying down. However, once asleep our muscles in the throat relax and the upper airway narrows. If the tonsils are too large, the narrowing of the airway will result in complete blockage. Apnea is the result. Repeated apnea results in sleep apnea syndrome.

There are other problems that occur in the upper airway. A small jaw (micrognathia) may cause obstruction of the airway. Small jaws are seen in advanced rheumatoid arthritis and some other conditions. These unfortunate individuals may develop apneas and sleep apnea syndrome as their arthritis progresses.

Obesity

Obesity can cause sleep apnea syndrome. Excessively obese people commonly have apneas and hypopneas and suffer from sleep apnea syndrome. Less severe obesity may or may not be associated with sleep apnea. The mechanisms for the apnea in these patients are similar to those in the patients with idiopathic sleep apnea. As sleep occurs, the airway narrows with relaxation. The airway size will be reduced in an obese person as fat in the palate and throat reduces the airway opening. In addition, body positions during sleep are limited because of their body size. The normal relaxation of the airway during sleep and the narrow airway together result in blockage.

Idiopathic Obstructive Sleep Apnea

Idiopathic obstructive sleep apnea accounts for sleep apnea syndrome in most patients. In these patients there is no medical problem causing the obstruction and no reason for the blockage of air can be identified. Excessive relaxation of the muscles of the throat is thought to result in collapse of the airway that blocks breathing. The site of the obstruction varies but can be either at the base of the tongue or at the soft palate and uvula.

It needs to be emphasized that idiopathic obstructive sleep apnea includes over 90% of patients with the syndrome. No identifiable specific cause can be found in most patients with sleep apnea syndrome.

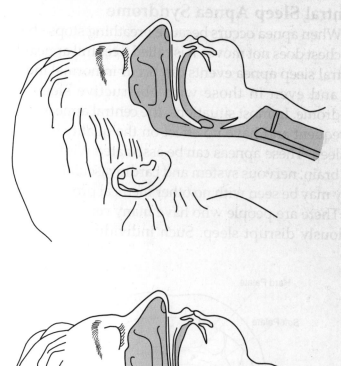

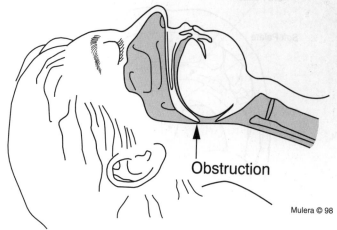

Obstruction

Mulera © 98

Obstruction of Airway
in Idiopathic Obstructive Sleep Apnea

The upper panel shows a reclining person during sleep, with no problems in the airway. When the airway muscles relax, the tongue and the palate close against the back of the pharynx blocking the airway as seen in the lower panel.

Figure 9-1

Central Sleep Apnea Syndrome

When apnea occurs because breathing stops - because the chest does not move - it is called a central apnea. These central sleep apnea events can occur in normal individuals and even in those with obstructive sleep apnea syndrome. In most situations, the central apneas are very infrequent and have no effect on the quality or quantity of sleep. These apneas can be associated with diseases of the brain, nervous system and cardiovascular system. Or, they may be seen with no other medical problem present.

There are people who have many central apneas that seriously disrupt sleep. Such individuals will develop

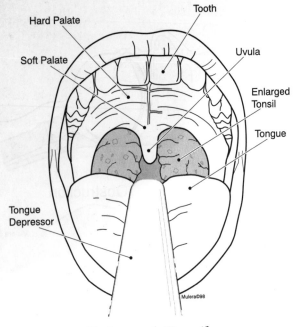

Enlarged Tonsils

Enlarged tonsils can cause intermittent obstruction of the upper airway and lead to Sleep Apnea Syndrome.

Figure 9-2

sleep apnea syndrome from the central apneas. Central sleep apnea as a cause of illness is very unusual and it can be difficult to treat.

COMPLICATIONS OF UNTREATED SLEEP APNEA SYNDROME

The effects of untreated sleep apnea syndrome can be drastic. While our understanding of the disease is still progressing, many of its effects are known. It is a serious disease and can result in death and prolonged illness.

Patients with sleep apnea have more heart attacks, sudden deaths, strokes and irregular heartbeats than do people who do not have sleep apnea syndrome. It is speculated that the severe drop in blood oxygen levels during apnea may be one reason for these problems as a result of the stress it places upon the heart.

Hypertension can result from sleep apnea. It has been estimated that about one-third of patients with sleep apnea syndrome have an elevated blood pressure and one-third of patients with hypertension have sleep apnea syndrome. When sleep apnea syndrome has not been treated, high blood pressure can be extremely difficult to treat and control.

Patients with the most severe cases of sleep apnea syndrome can have problems with the blood vessels in their lungs. Repeated drops in the amount of oxygen in the blood may cause muscle spasms in the arterial blood vessels to the lung - the pulmonary arteries. As the spasms occur more frequently, the blood vessels may become fixed in a narrow condition. This will produce pulmonary hypertension which is high blood pressure in the pulmonary arteries. This special form of high blood pressure can stress the right side of the heart and result in right heart failure.

The brain can be affected in various ways by problems with blood pressure. Strokes are more frequent in untreated sleep apnea and also in patients where blood pressure is high. There is evidence that patients with sleep apnea have problems with thinking. Their mental abilities appear to suffer. Memory becomes poor. From studies of sleep apnea patients in the sleep laboratory, periods of low blood oxygen can be seen to affect the electrical recordings (the electroencephalogram) of brain waves. Brain cells are known to be very dependent upon oxygen. Consequently, low blood oxygen rapidly affects brain cell function.

One of the most serious effects of sleep apnea syndrome is excessive sleepiness. People with sleep apnea syndrome have a high rate of serious accidents. And frequently, those accidents involve automobiles and result in death or serious injury to the patient and to others.

TESTS USED FOR
SLEEP APNEA SYNDROME

The tests used to diagnose sleep apnea syndrome can vary depending on the physician and the suspected problem. A sleep study is required to diagnose and document the problem and its severity. The majority of sleep studies (called polysomnograms) are performed through a sleep laboratory.

A sleep study measures changes that occur during sleep. The number of arousals (partial awakenings from sleep) that occur are measured. The number of apneas, hypopneas and movements of the limbs are measured. From these measurements, the quality and quantity of

COMPLICATIONS OF UNTREATED SLEEP APNEA SYNDROME

These medical problems occur significantly more often in patients with Sleep Apnea Syndrome.

- ➤ Sudden Death
- ➤ Heart Attacks
- ➤ Heart Rhythm Abnormalities
- ➤ Hypertension
- ➤ Pulmonary Hypertension
- ➤ Heart Failure
- ➤ Strokes
- ➤ Decreased Mental Capacity
- ➤ Excessive Sleepiness
- ➤ Serious Accidents
- ➤ Death from Accidents

sleep can be estimated, the effects of respirations and leg movements on sleep are seen and, the rhythm of the heart is observed.

Some of the important numbers obtained are the indexes. An index is the number of times an hour something happens. The *Apnea Index* is the number of apneas recorded per hour. The *Hypopnea Index* is the number of hypopneas per hour. The *Apnea/Hypopnea Index* is a combination of the two, the number of apneas plus the number of hypopneas per hour.

The severity of the disease is established from several factors. The most important is the apnea/hypopnea index. Index levels less than 15 are mild. Indexes between 15-30 are considered moderate. Indexes of greater than

TESTS FOR SLEEP APNEA SYNDROME

SLEEP STUDY (POLYSOMNOGRAM)

Measures
- Quality and quantity of sleep
- Respiratory and cardiac events
- Limb movements

Information obtained
- Sleep stages
- Sleep time and depth
- Awakenings and arousals
- Cardiac rhythm
- Oxygen levels
- Indexes (events per hour)

MULTIPLE SLEEP LATENCY TESTING (MSLT)
- Measures sleepiness
- Information obtained
  - Time to fall asleep
  - Sleep stages

30 are considered to be severe. Other important factors in determining severity of sleep apnea are the length of each apnea, the size of the drop of oxygen levels in the blood, the number of arousals, the cardiac rhythm that occurs during apneas, and the degree of daytime symptoms.

Daytime symptoms may be measured by performing a Multiple Sleep Latency Test (MSLT). The test, usually performed the day following a sleep study, measures sleepiness.

TEMPORARY SLEEP APNEA SYNDROME

Sleep apnea can cause problems intermittently and for short periods of time in apparently normal individuals. Only when sleep events occur in significant numbers do they affect a person and cause the problems of sleep apnea syndrome. Physicians are still debating the differences between normal sleep and abnormal sleep, but one fact is clear. There are apparently normal people who develop the signs and symptoms of sleep apnea syndrome in certain situations. These situations also will make someone with very mild sleep apnea or patients with significant sleep apnea, worse.

The most common situation that worsens breathing problems during sleep is the common head cold. Blocking the nose with mucus, the cold causes difficulty breathing through the upper airway. This difficulty in breathing will increase the tendency for blockage of the upper airway.

Alcohol causes increased relaxation of the muscles in the airway. This relaxation produces more obstruction to breathing and more sleep disturbance. Sedatives, muscle relaxers, pain relievers, and other medications work similarly to alcohol, causing more breathing problems. Antihistamines dry out the mucus membranes of the airway. Dry membranes tend to stick together and may cause more breathing problems during sleep.

After undergoing surgery, patients may be required to sleep on their backs, take medications that affect their breathing, or have problems with their noses. Any of these events can affect or worsen any sleep disordered breathing problem.

As a result of common colds, medications, alcohol, or surgery, sleep apnea may be made worse, or a snorer may be converted to someone with sleep apnea. After the cold clears, the medication or alcohol wears off, or the patient returns to a normal sleeping position, the person's sleep will return to its previous state. During these temporary episodes of sleep apnea, treatment is usually not required, however, in some selected situations it may be needed for a short period of time.

POSITIONAL SLEEP APNEA

In some individuals, sleep apnea only occurs when sleeping on the back. When they sleep on their sides or stomachs, they breathe normally. The symptoms they have and the problems they develop depend upon their sleeping positions. If they are able to sleep without lying on their backs, they may be free of problems.

A person with no symptoms or signs of sleep apnea may have problems with sleep apnea if forced to sleep on his back. For example, after some surgeries a patient must stay on his back for a period of time. Or, problems with arthritis or an injury may make it difficult to sleep on the side or stomach.

The natural movements during sleep always result in some time sleeping on our backs. When a positional sleep apnea problem is present, the more time spent on the back, the more likely symptoms or problems will develop.

Sleep Apnea Syndrome
CHAPTER SUMMARY

SLEEP APNEA SYNDROME

The disease produced by repeated disturbance of sleep by respiratory events such as apnea or hypopnea

A common medical disorder occurring in all ages and both sexes, but more commonly in men and the elderly

SYMPTOMS

➤ The symptoms vary considerably but are usually related to daytime sleepiness.

SIGNS OF THE DISEASE

➤ The major signs which suggest sleep apnea are snoring and having apnea which is observed during sleep.

CAUSES OF SLEEP APNEA SYNDROME

➤ Obesity
➤ Low thyroid hormone levels
➤ Obstruction of the upper airway
➤ Idiopathic Obstructive (no known cause)
   —The most common situation
➤ Central Sleep Apnea
   —A rare form of sleep apnea

(continued on next page)

Sleep Apnea Syndrome
CHAPTER SUMMARY *(continued)*

COMPLICATIONS OF SLEEP APNEA SYNDROME
- Hypertension
- Heart Attacks
- Sleepiness
- Pulmonary Hypertension
- Memory Problems
- Irregular Heartbeats
- Strokes
- Sudden Deaths
- Accidents

TESTS FOR SLEEP APNEA
- Sleep study (polysomnogram)
  —measures the quality and quantity of sleep and breathing
- Multiple sleep latency testing (MSLT)
  —measures the degree of sleepiness during the day

TEMPORARY SLEEP APNEA
- Brought on by common cold, medications, alcohol, or sleeping position
- Resolves when the cause is taken away

POSITIONAL SLEEP APNEA
- Sleep apnea which occurs in only one position

Chapter Ten

Treatment of Sleep Apnea Syndrome

There are a limited number of ways to treat sleep apnea syndrome. How the treatment is selected depends upon the cause of the sleep apnea, the severity of the disease, the physician's experience, the patient's preference, and to some degree, who pays for the treatment.

Sometimes the severity of disease determines the type and urgency of treatment. If severe sleep apnea syndrome is identified, treatment may be needed on an urgent basis. If the sleep apnea is affecting other medical conditions such as heart disease, rapid treatment may be required. More commonly, sleep apnea syndrome can be evaluated and treated routinely.

There are general considerations that may benefit anyone with sleep problems. Good sleep habits are helpful and even more important when suffering from sleep apnea syndrome. Allowing adequate sleeping time and practicing good sleep habits are very important and can lead to improvement in the quality and quantity of sleep.

When obesity is associated with sleep apnea syndrome, weight loss can be very beneficial. If the obese patient is able to lose a significant amount of weight (approximately 10%), improvement and sometimes resolution of the sleep apnea may occur. Weight reduction, while a very desirable form of therapy, is often extremely difficult to achieve.

It is important to keep adequately hydrated, since dryness aggravates the obstructive events. Drinking an adequate amount of water is the best hydration.

All medications taken for any condition should be reviewed once a diagnosis of sleep apnea syndrome is made. There are medications that can aggravate the condition. With sleep apnea syndrome, it is important to avoid drugs that cause drowsiness. They may increase the frequency and severity of the sleep apnea. Medications that cause dryness may increase problems with the obstructions. Antihistamines should be avoided. Alcohol may produce mild sleep apnea or make existing sleep apnea much worse.

TREATMENT OF SPECIFIC CONDITIONS

If a specific cause can be identified, the sleep apnea may be cured by correcting the problem.

Hypothyroidism is a treatable cause of sleep apnea syndrome. Patients with low thyroid hormone levels are treated with thyroid hormone replacement. The replacement is carried out slowly over several months in order to allow the body to adjust to the new levels. When the thyroid hormone levels return to normal, which may require a year or more, the sleep apnea is usually completely corrected. Often, during the months it takes to correct the low levels, other forms of treatment for the sleep apnea syndrome may be needed.

Another example of a specific cause of sleep apnea syndrome is enlarged tonsils. In this situation, removal of the tonsils usually cures the problem. Before and after surgery (tonsillectomy) other forms of treatment may be required on a temporary basis.

TREATMENT OF IDIOPATHIC OBSTRUCTIVE SLEEP APNEA SYNDROME

As we have learned in the preceding chapter, the cause of idiopathic obstructive sleep apnea syndrome is unknown. The current theory to explain the obstruction in these patients is over-relaxation of the throat muscles during sleep. Time and research will determine the cause or causes, but for now, a number of treatments directed at preventing the apneas to improve sleep are available. While many have been tried in this disorder, the ideal treatment is yet to be identified. General statements can be made about the value of each technique, but it should be remembered, each individual may respond differently.

MEDICATIONS AND SLEEP APNEA SYNDROME

A number of drugs have been used to treat sleep apnea syndrome, but with only marginal benefit. While medications cannot cure sleep apnea, they may serve as aids in treatment.

Some of these medications include drugs to stimulate breathing. Hormone preparations such as progesterone and respiratory stimulants such as theophylline are examples. These drugs stimulate respiration and can reduce the numbers of apneas and hypopneas in some patients.

There are medications that promote mucus flow and moisture in the upper airway. These medications may reduce dryness in the throat. A moist throat helps prevent some apneas and hypopneas. One example of these medications is guaifenesin. Water is the best moisturizer. Drinking an adequate amount of water each day, six to eight, 8 ounce glasses, may help decrease the severity of sleep apnea.

Oxygen is a drug. It seems logical that oxygen might help patients with sleep apnea syndrome. Unfortunately, it usually does not help. Taken during sleep, oxygen may actually make the apneas last longer. Some patients do benefit from oxygen though a physician will have to decide for each case and repeated study of oxygen levels during sleep may be required.

Stimulants may be used by some physicians as aids to staying awake in some selected patients. These drugs are used primarily for the treatment of narcolepsy and their use in sleep apnea syndrome is mostly limited to those who have failed other therapies directed at correcting the apneas.

DEVICES

The majority of patients with sleep apnea syndrome are treated with these non-invasive forms of therapy. They have been successful and are the most common mode of treatment used. They include positional devices, dental appliances, and positive air pressure given through a mask over the nose.

Positional Therapy

Sleep apnea problems may occur more frequently while sleeping on the back than on the sides. Sometimes apneas and hypopneas occur only when sleeping on the back. In these special situations the sleep disorder can be corrected by not allowing sleep while lying on the back.

The most common way to prevent sleeping while lying on the back is to attach some device to the back of a nightshirt that is worn while sleeping. If the person rolls onto his back, the object on the back of the shirt will cause discomfort and the person will then roll back onto his side to resume sleeping.

The easiest way to make a positional nightshirt requires a tee shirt, a pair of large socks, four small safety pins and two cans of tennis balls. The socks are filled with the tennis balls and pinned to the back of the tee shirt. The shirt is worn while sleeping.

Positional therapy is an effective treatment for sleep apnea that occurs only when sleeping on the back.

Dental Appliances

Dental appliances are used to keep the jaw in a forward position. They are custom-made for each individual and are worn while sleeping. Their value has been confirmed by scientific study and they can be an effective treatment for mild sleep apnea syndrome. Unfortunately, with moderate or severe disease, dental appliances are not as successful. After an appliance has been made, a period of sleep will need to be observed while using the appliance to measure its effectiveness.

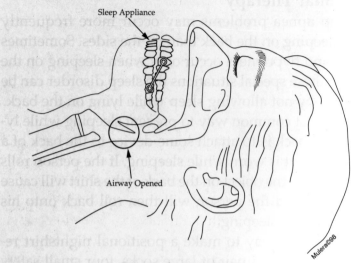

Sleep Appliance

Airway Opened

Mulera©98

Dental Appliance

A number of dental appliances have been developed to treat obstructive sleep apnea. The appliance is worn at night and fits over the teeth. The jaw is held forward by the appliance which keeps the airway open.

Figure 10-1

Nasal Continuous Positive Airway Pressure (Nasal CPAP)

Nasal CPAP (pronounced nasal see pap) is the most widely used form of therapy for obstructive sleep apnea and it is the most effective. It can eliminate the breathing problem during sleep 98% of the time.

The advantages of nasal CPAP are that it is easy to use, does not require surgery and can be replaced when something better comes along. On the other hand, a mask must be worn each night, nasal dryness often occurs, and the machine to generate the positive pressure must run all night.

A nasal CPAP machine passes air continuously into the nose to keep the air pressure in the nose and throat higher than normal. The positive air pressure keeps the throat from collapsing and obstructing during sleep.

Air is passed into the nose through a mask. Several types and sizes of masks are available, but all the masks function the same. Getting a mask which is comfortable and fits properly is a very important part of nasal CPAP therapy.

The air pressure required to keep the airway open is generated by a nasal CPAP machine. This machine sits on the bedside table and generates airflow that passes through a tube to the mask. The mask and tube are attached with a swivel so that any sleeping position can be achieved.

The pressure required to treat sleep apnea is different for each patient with the disease. It is determined by undergoing a sleep study while wearing the mask. The pressure can be adjusted during the study to make sure the breathing problem is corrected.

In some individuals, oxygen may be needed in addition to nasal CPAP in order to correct the breathing problem. During the sleep study with nasal CPAP, the need for oxygen can be evaluated.

Bilevel Positive Airway Pressure

Bilevel PAP is a form of nasal CPAP. When using bilevel PAP, the air pressure is different during inspiration and expiration. During CPAP, the same airway pressure is maintained all the time. Bilevel systems are used most commonly in patients with sleep apnea when there is a need for a very high pressure. With bilevel PAP, the mask and tubing are the same as used with CPAP, only the pressure machine is changed.

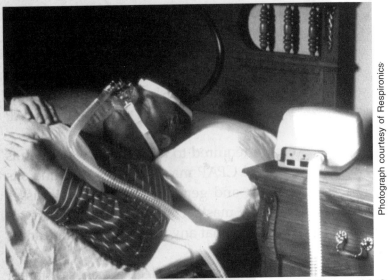

Photograph courtesy of Respironics

Nasal CPAP

Figure 10-2

Wearing a mask allows someone with sleep apnea to sleep normally. Many masks and machines are available.

Continuously Self-Adjusting Nasal CPAP

This is the newest form of CPAP and it has been designed to be self-adjusting. Few studies have been reported utilizing this form of therapy and clinical experience is limited.

QUESTIONS AND PROBLEMS WITH NASAL CPAP

The most frequent problem reported with nasal CPAP is nose dryness. The amount of air needed to maintain the correct pressure can dry out the nasal passages, but the nose usually adapts over time. There are some steps that can help. Drinking plenty of water is advantageous. Saline nasal spray may be used before bedtime and in the

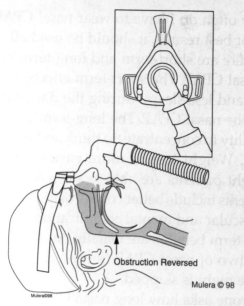

Obstruction Reversed

Mulera © 98

Mulera©98

Constant Positive Airway Pressure

Positive airway pressure is delivered to the airway through a mask usually worn over the nose. It holds the pharynx open with air pressure.

Figure 10-3

morning. A mucolytic medication such as guaifenesin may be prescribed by your physician. For persistent problems with dryness, a humidifier may be added to the nasal CPAP machine.

Individuals who have problems with sinus conditions, such as sinusitis or allergic nasal problems, will note more difficulties with these problems when they are on nasal CPAP. Any difficulties should be brought to the attention of your physician. Usually, these can be prevented or treated satisfactorily. Nasal CPAP may have to be discontinued briefly and in some cases a different form of treatment used.

"How often do I have to wear nasal CPAP?" is often asked. For best results, it should be used all night, every night. There are short-term and long-term benefits from using nasal CPAP. The short-term effects are mostly being alert and less sleepy during the day after the nights you use the nasal CPAP. The long-term effects include a better ability to concentrate, to think and to perform mental tasks. Weight loss is more easily achieved when overweight patients are able to sleep well. Other long-term benefits include better control of high blood pressure, cardiovascular and mental complications of sleep apnea.

Long-term benefits are usually not lost by skipping a night or two of nasal CPAP. Short-term benefits are lost when one night is skipped.

Everyone asks how long nasal CPAP will be needed. It will be required until there is a change in your condition or your sleep apnea. For example, if a significant weight loss occurs, you may not need nasal CPAP. If a new treatment is developed for sleep apnea, you may be able to quit using your nasal CPAP.

Some people are unable to sleep well after starting nasal CPAP. Many times this is related to the sleep habits developed when suffering from being too sleepy. Patients with sleep apnea often learn to drink caffeinated beverages to fight off sleepiness. When they start to use nasal CPAP, the caffeine that they have been taking begins to keep them awake at night. A review of your personal habits and any medication taken is needed when treatment for sleep apnea is started.

SURGICAL TREATMENT OF SLEEP APNEA

The first treatment for sleep apnea syndrome was surgical. Now there are several procedures which may be used in appropriate situations.

The characteristics of all surgical procedures include the need for anesthesia, risk of complications, a permanent change in anatomy, and a need for retesting after the wounds have healed. It is unfortunate, but often the sleep apnea will need treatment by other means — usually nasal CPAP and sometimes a tracheostomy — before and after the surgery.

Tracheostomy

A tracheostomy procedure is the creation of an opening between the windpipe (trachea) and the air outside the throat. Although it was the first procedure performed to treat sleep apnea syndrome, now it is rarely used as a permanent treatment. A tracheostomy corrects obstruc-

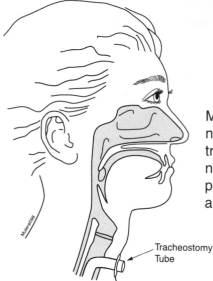

Tracheostomy

Making an opening in the neck through the skin into the trachea eliminates sleep apnea. Unfortunately the procedure is only suitable for a few individuals.

Tracheostomy Tube

Figure 10-4

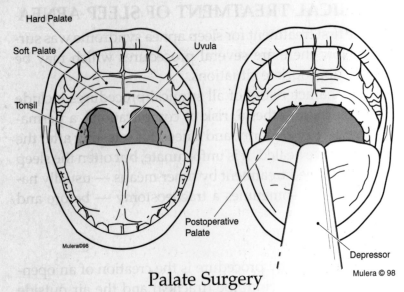

Hard Palate

Soft Palate

Tonsil

Uvula

Postoperative
Palate

Depressor

Mulera©98

Mulera © 98

Palate Surgery

Surgical removal of a portion of the palate and uvula may benefit some patients with sleep apnea syndrome. The procedure demonstrated here shows a throat before and after a uvulopalatopharyngoplasty.

Figure 10-5

tive sleep apnea 100% of the time. Unfortunately, there are significant side effects and numerous complications that can develop from a tracheostomy with time. The side effects and complications are often more serious than the problems of sleep apnea syndrome and as a result, the procedure is used only in selected cases. It may be needed to temporarily treat apneas during surgery for sleep apnea or during other major surgeries.

Uvulopalatopharyngoplasty

This is the surgical removal of the uvula and portions of the palate and pharyngeal wall, which are tissues that can cause obstruction in sleep apnea. It is performed under general anesthesia in an operating room and may require several days in the hospital.

It is an effective treatment for snoring, but it is not an excellent treatment for sleep apnea syndrome. It can correct sleep apnea in about one-third of cases. It can improve but not correct sleep apnea in another third, and in the last third, it has no effect. As a result, about one-half of patients with sleep apnea syndrome who have a uvulopalatopharyngoplasty still need nightly treatment with some other form of therapy.

Unfortunately, physicians cannot clearly identify the patients whose sleep apnea will benefit from this type of surgery. As a result, patients who have surgery need to be retested with a sleep study following the procedure. The main sign of sleep apnea syndrome, snoring, will usually disappear after surgery.

Laser-assisted uvulopalatoplasty (LAUP)

LAUP is a limited form of a uvulopalatopharyngoplasty. It may be performed in a physician's office as an outpatient under local anesthesia using a laser to remove tissue. Only the uvula and a portion of the palate are removed. This procedure is widely available. Like the uvulopalatopharyngoplasty, a LAUP does an excellent job of treating snoring but is not usually an effective treatment for sleep apnea syndrome.

Radiofrequency Palatoplasty

This procedure shrinks the size of the soft palate. A small probe is inserted into the soft palate after local anesthesia has been given. A low frequency radiowave is generated from the probe and damages the tissue of the palate. As the tissue heals, it scars and retracts the soft palate, reducing its size.

The procedure is performed in physicians' offices. It has proven somewhat successful in the treatment of snoring, but has no proven ability to treat obstructive sleep apnea.

Tonsillectomy

When obstruction is caused by enlarged tonsils or adenoids, surgical removal may cure the sleep apnea syndrome.

Nasal surgery

In a limited number of individuals, nasal obstruction contributes to sleep apnea. Surgical removal of the nasal obstruction and correction of deviated septums may benefit some of these individuals.

Additional procedures

There are a number of additional procedures that are performed on selected patients. These surgical procedures move a portion of the throat, jaw or cranium to open the airway and prevent sleep apnea. In the appropriate person, these surgeries can be successful. They are major procedures, have risk, and require general anesthesia. The procedures are considered in patients who have significant sleep apnea and in whom other forms of therapy have failed. X-rays of the head must be evaluated as they help select candidates for these procedures. The procedures are usually performed in steps with healing between the surgeries. After each surgery, sleep testing is required to establish whether the sleep apnea was corrected.

Hyoidplasty is used in selected patients with a small narrow hypopharynx. A brace placed on the hyoid bone expands, stabilizes it and results in opening the hypopharynx.

Other procedures include hyoid suspension, mandibular advancement and maxillary plate advancement. In

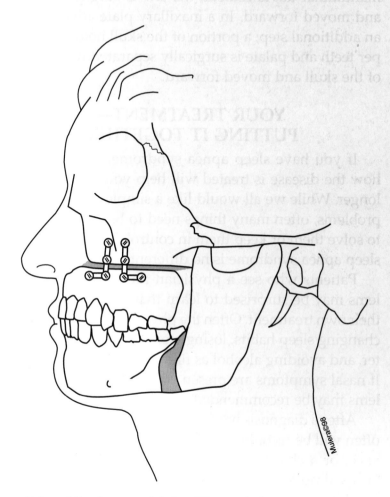

Mandibular and Maxillary Advancement

This illustration shows, in the shaded area, how the mandible (jaw) and maxilla (upper jaw) can be advanced by separating them from the rest of the bone, moved forward and secured in place.

Figure 10-6

mandibular advancement, the jaw is surgically broken
and moved forward. In a maxillary plate advancement,
an additional step, a portion of the skull holding the upper teeth and palate is surgically separated from the rest
of the skull and moved forward.

YOUR TREATMENT— PUTTING IT TOGETHER

If you have sleep apnea syndrome, understanding
how the disease is treated will help you live better and
longer. While we all would like a simple answer for our
problems, often many things need to be done over time
to solve them or keep them in control. The treatment for
sleep apnea syndrome is no different.

Patients who see a physician for sleep apnea problems may be surprised to learn that they have a role in
their own treatment. Often the physician will recommend
changing sleep habits, losing weight, drinking more water, and avoiding alcohol as first steps in their treatment.
If nasal symptoms are present, treatment for those problems may be recommended.

After a diagnosis has been confirmed, other treatment
often will be recommended. Nasal CPAP, a dental appliance, or a change in sleep position might be needed.
Surgical options may be discussed. The importance of
good sleep habits, weight loss and other activities are
usually reviewed.

As time passes, the physician will review your
progress or lack of progress. Side effects of the treatment
can be dealt with and new treatments tried if needed.

Treatment requires your work and cooperation. The more
effort you put into it, the better you will feel and live.

Treatment of Obstructive Sleep Apnea
CHAPTER SUMMARY

GENERAL MEASURES
- Good sleep habits
- Weight loss
- Medication review

TREATMENT OF SPECIFIC CONDITIONS
- Corrects sleep apnea
- Examples include hypothyroidism and enlarged tonsils
- May require other temporary treatments for apneas

TREATMENT OF IDIOPATHIC OBSTRUCTIVE SLEEP APNEA
- Cause or causes unknown
- Treatment directed at apneas

MEDICATIONS — Not very helpful

DEVICES
- Positional - For apnea while sleeping on back
- Dental Appliances - For mild sleep apnea
- Nasal constant positive air pressure—Nasal CPAP
  - —Most common form of treatment
  - —For mild to severe problems

SURGERY
- A number of procedures are available
- Procedures are selected upon an individual basis

YOUR TREATMENT— WORK FOR YOURSELF WITH YOUR PHYSICIAN

SECTION IV

COMMON SLEEP
PROBLEMS
AND DISORDERS

A few sleep disorders account for the majority of sleep problems. This section covers those which you are most likely to experience.

Section IV Common Sleep Problems and Disorders

Chapter Eleven

Sleep Habits and Their Problems

SLEEP HABITS

Habits are a part of us. We find ways to do things in life that are comfortable and easy. These ways of doing things when repeated often become a part of our lives. They become habits. We do many things out of habit. The many habits we do automatically and the activities we do by choice have a big impact on the quality of our sleep. Sometimes, changing the things we do can improve our sleep.

There are many factors under our control that can influence the quality of our sleep and our well-being during the day. Our choices of bedtimes and the length of time we allow ourselves to sleep are examples. The activities we do and when we do them, the foods and drugs we take, and our sleeping environment are things we determine by choice.

Timing Sleep

The ability to feel rested and full of energy after a night's sleep depends on many things. Most importantly is the total time of sleep during the night.

We have individual requirements for sleep which averages about eight hours. If we go to bed at midnight and awaken to an alarm at 6:00, we have only allowed six hours to sleep. For most, it will not be enough. If we continue to sleep only six hours a night, each day we will become progressively more fatigued. Usually, after several days, we sleep longer and catch up. Our weekend "sleep in" is the result of this behavior.

Bedtime and the amount of time allowed for sleep are choices we make. They can be changed. They are often changed because of social, work, personal or family obligations. We choose to do something else rather than sleep. We stay up late. We get up earlier.

To be refreshed and restored for a new day, even high quality sleep needs adequate time. While we cannot always allow the amount of time needed for sleep, we can try.

It is particularly important for someone who has problems with sleep to have an adequate amount of time to sleep. The sleep time should start at an appropriate time of the day for our bodies' desire, our work requirements and our social schedules.

The ideal approach is to have a fixed bedtime and a fixed time to awaken. The more you are able to sleep the planned time, the more refreshing your sleep will be.

Sleeping Environment

Sleep is better in a dark, quiet, comfortable place. Light affects our sleep. The eyelids do not block out all light, and light stimulates us and our brains through our eyes. It is difficult to sleep in bright light. Darkness helps us sleep well.

Noise, like light, affects our sleep. Noise of a changing loudness or changing pitch can disturb sleep. The body can screen out much noise when sleep is needed, but the quieter the sleep space, the better the sleep.

Some people say they sleep better with some noise present, a radio or television is typical. White noise, background noise of relatively constant loudness and pitch, may help some to sleep better. It filters out other noise which might contrast sharply with silence when the white sound is not present. Many sound machines are available commercially.

Sleep specialists discourage the use of radio and television for a source of white sound. The problem with them as a source for sound is the content and lack of control over volume. The mind and body may sleep, but what they hear and how they react are not fully known or understood. If you must use some noise to help you sleep, a sound machine or recorded music are both preferable to television or radio broadcasts.

The room must not only be quiet and dark, it must be comfortable as well. The temperature should be pleasant in all seasons. The bed should be comfortable and the mattress replaced regularly. Most sleep better when the room is clean and the linens are fresh.

Activities and Sleep

There are activities that can interfere with our sleep. Many activities stimulate our bodies through the nervous and endocrine systems. Some activities decrease our need for sleep.

Exercise causes our bodies to come to full alertness. The stimulation of exercise releases epinephrine into our systems. Sleep is almost impossible immediately after exercise. As time passes, the effect wears off and the ability to sleep returns. Therefore, exercise should be performed several hours before bedtime.

The response to exercise can be produced in other situations. The body can be fooled into thinking it is about to exercise or should be ready to exercise. An adventure movie or video can fool your body into thinking that you need to be ready to participate in the action. Your body will think that you are going to exercise, so several hours will be needed for it to be ready for sleep.

A well-written book can have the same effect on many people. A fast-moving adventure novel is hard to put down. It can be difficult to sleep even after one puts aside the book, because the body is ready for action.

Some of our need for sleep is determined by what we do during the day. If we are physically active, we need more sleep. If we are physically inactive, we need less.

We only need a certain amount of sleep. If we sleep some during the day, we may sleep less at night. For example, after a nap we will need less sleep at night. It may be more difficult to go to sleep and stay asleep if you nap during the day.

Pre-Sleep Ritual

Sleep comes most easily when an established pattern of events occurs before trying to go to sleep. The steps performed getting ready for bed have been called the pre-sleep ritual.

Typical steps that could be considered part of the ritual might include preparing the house for the night, having a snack, preparing the pets, bathing, brushing teeth, setting an alarm clock, and turning off the lights. Depending upon the person, one or more of these steps may be part of their pre-sleep ritual.

The consistent repetition of the steps each night makes the sequence of steps into a ritual. The more consistently the ritual is carried out the more calming the effect. A consistent ritual promotes sleep onset and improves the quality of sleep.

Food and Drugs

Eating and what we eat affect our sleep. After a meal, our bodies focus on the digestion and storing of our food which often makes us feel sleepy. Typically, the larger the meal, the more tired and sleepy we feel. An excessively large meal will result in disturbed sleep. When we eat a meal near bedtime, we increase the likelihood that our sleep will be affected. Sleep may come on easily, but the sleep will not be good sleep. It will not be refreshing.

Certain types of food can affect our sleep. Each of us has foods we have learned do not agree with our digestive systems. Eating foods that do not agree with us results in aftereffects. If eaten before bedtime, they may affect our sleep.

There is some evidence that a small snack at bedtime, or just before, improves the quality of sleep.

The products we drink can play a major role in our sleep. Drinks with caffeine and drinks with alcohol both significantly affect sleep.

Coffee, tea, and now sodas, have been in the diet of much of the world for several centuries. The caffeine in some of these products produces a stimulating effect that most of us use to start our day and boost us at other times during the day when we feel fatigued. Our use of these products can affect our sleep. Often our use increases gradually over time and can reach levels that interfere with sleep on a regular basis.

Caffeine may delay sleep onset and reduce the quality of sleep. Older individuals are more sensitive to caffeine than are the young. If you are having a sleep problem, the caffeine in your diet should be reduced or totally eliminated.

Alcohol makes most people sleepy. It speeds sleep onset. Unfortunately, the quality of sleep usually is poor after drinking alcohol and individuals with sleep problems should restrict its use or avoid it altogether.

Medications interfere with sleep. If you take drugs regularly and are having a sleep problem, review your prescriptions carefully.

Sleep Habits
CHAPTER SUMMARY

TIMING SLEEP
- Allow enough time (usually eight hours)
- Keep the same bedtime and awake time each day

SLEEPING ENVIRONMENT
- Dark, quiet and pleasant
- Clean and comfortable bed
- Background noise sometimes helpful

ACTIVITIES NEAR BEDTIME
- No exercise near bedtime
- No stimulating television
- No eating in bed
- No stimulating reading

PRE-SLEEP ACTIVITIES
- Establish a pre-sleep routine

FOOD AND DRUGS
- No meals near bedtime
- Avoid caffeine
- Avoid excessive alcohol
- Review medications carefully

SLEEP AND HABITS
- Attention to sleep-related habits can enhance the quality and quantity of sleep

Chapter 12

Insomnia

Going to sleep or staying asleep can be a problem for all of us at one time or another. Worrying about our job or loved ones, an illness or injury, and the results of an overly generous meal all can cause problems sleeping. These difficulties are usually brief and self-limited, and normally the reason is obvious and easy to manage. When the reason is unclear or the problem remains for days or weeks, further information or professional help may be needed.

A large number of problems can produce symptoms of insomnia. In these situations, the difficulty going to sleep represents a secondary effect from these problems and treatment directed at correcting them usually results in better sleep. The list of reasons for insomnia is extensive.

Unfortunately, many people who complain of insomnia do not have an easily recognized problem that causes it. This is frequently the case when the difficulty sleeping has been present for months or years. In these individuals, the sleeping difficulty has become the problem. This situation is called psychophysiological insomnia and also includes difficulty brought on by anxiety and stress. Let's look at each type separately.

Causes of Insomnia

There are many reasons for insomnia and many problems cause it. Excessive eating and drinking make sleep difficult. Excessive caffeine and chronic alcohol use affect the ability to go to sleep and stay asleep. A hot room or hunger pangs can interrupt sleep. Insomnia can be the result of medical conditions as bothersome as the common cold, as irritating as the pain of a sprained ankle, or as distressing as a diagnosis of cancer. These situations are usually obvious to both patient and physician and control of the medical condition helps improve sleep. If the condition cannot be improved, treatment with medications may improve symptoms.

Insomnia can be the result of psychiatric illnesses. Depression and schizophrenia are typical examples. Sleep apnea and other sleep disorders such as periodic limb movements can result in poor sleep. Generally, sleep improves with the identification and treatment of these problems.

Medications used to treat illnesses may interfere with sleep. A variety of medications from antibiotics to antidepressants can cause difficulty going to sleep and staying asleep. When difficulty in sleeping develops, any medications taken for medical problems should be reviewed for a possible role.

Psychophysiologic Insomnia

Difficulty going to sleep and staying asleep can arise from our personal responses to life and its difficulties. While the exact reason may be obvious, many times it is

CAUSES OF TOO LITTLE SLEEP

➤ Psychophysiologic

➤ Drugs - Caffeine, Alcohol, Medications

➤ Medical Illnesses

➤ Environmental

➤ Perception

➤ Psychiatric

➤ Periodic Limb Movements

➤ Sleep Apnea

➤ Restless Legs

not, or there are many reasons working together. When social and personal interactions at work and at home result in problems sleeping they are classified as psychophysiologic.

The stresses of modern life frequently produce this form of insomnia. When difficulty with sleep has developed within the past two or three months, the event or events leading to it are usually clear, although sometimes another person or a professional may have to help identify them. Identification is important. Knowing why sleep does not come easily takes away fears of a more serious illness. It also helps by allowing the person to focus on placing into practice good sleep habits. Medications may be needed to help sleep onset, but are of only temporary value. Most symptoms of insomnia resolve when the reasons for them goes away.

SHORT-TERM / CHRONIC INSOMNIA

INSOMNIA — The symptoms of not sleeping well. The perception of not getting enough sleep. It is the difficulty of going to sleep and staying asleep.

SHORT-TERM INSOMNIA
➤ Usually secondary to a recognized problem
➤ Response to life and its difficulties
   —Result of stress or emotional turmoil
   —Result of medical problems

CHRONIC INSOMNIA
➤ Insomnia present for months or years
➤ May be a result of medical, psychiatric and sleep problems or their treatment
➤ Usually no cause apparent - not secondary

Unfortunately, problems with insomnia that persist for months and years can become serious and difficult to improve. These situations are called chronic insomnia.

Chronic Insomnia

Insomnia that has been present for a long time (months to years) is often a difficult problem for both patients and physicians. Frequently in these situations, the events that started the problems with sleep have gone away and only the difficulty sleeping remains. It cannot be associated with personal, medical or psychiatric problems. There is no specific cause identifiable for the insomnia and no simple answer to the problem exists. In these situations, improvement requires patient effort and understanding.

Of course, long-standing medical, psychiatric and sleep problems or their treatments can lead to chronic difficulties with sleeping. In these situations, treatment for insomnia is best directed at those problems and success is dependent on the ability to treat them. Long-standing sleep difficulty that is not secondary to other reasons or causes is called chronic insomnia and classified as psychophysiological.

Our understanding of chronic insomnia is limited. It is thought that whatever started the insomnia problem in these individuals disappeared long before they sought help. The insomnia becomes a part of their lives after its onset. Why? We are not sure, but there are several possible explanations.

Insomnia may go on and on for several reasons. Our habits contribute to how well we sleep. Many who suffer from chronic insomnia have personal habits that do not help them sleep. Actually, many habits keep us from sleeping well. Eating late, exercising late, drinking excessive alcohol, watching television in bed, and napping during the day all reduce the quality of sleep.

Once someone develops problems sleeping, they work harder at trying to sleep. The effect of trying to sleep better may backfire. The process of going to bed becomes dreaded. The steps preparing for bed lead to more alertness and more difficulty sleeping. As the effort to sleep intensifies, so do the problems with sleep. Problems sleeping become expected and then they occur.

There is another factor to be considered. How much sleep is really occurring? Patients with problems sleeping commonly underestimate the amount of time they actually sleep. Because they feel tired in the morning, have problems going to sleep, and have problems awakening during the night, their perception of the amount of sleep they obtain is shorter than the time they actually slept.

These three factors all contribute to the persistence of chronic insomnia: personal habits that disturb sleep, a dread of trying to sleep, and thinking they sleep less than they do.

Treatment of Chronic Insomnia

Treatment requires cooperation and understanding. It frequently improves problems with insomnia, but unfortunately, these conditions are often lifelong. The goal of treatment is to improve the quality of sleep for the person. Treatment is different for each person but directed at changing and improving the above three factors.

Since personal habits play a large role in our sleep, good habits improve sleep. The habits that can affect sleep are extensive. They are the subject of their own chapter in this book. Attention to these habits will improve sleep quality.

Insomnia does not cause illnesses or medical problems. Patients often become so involved with trying to sleep, their lives suffer. Not sleeping well is a cause for concern, but acceptance and adaptation play a major role in overcoming insomnia. Some of history's most productive people suffered from insomnia. If you have chronic insomnia, you are among good company. Is it possible to use some of your time in another way? Are you ready to start that novel? How many unfinished projects need attention?

Relaxation techniques may assist in going to sleep. Counting sheep, slow deep breathing or progressive muscle relaxation may be helpful. More details on these techniques can be found at your library, through a book store, or from your physician or sleep specialist.

A technique called stimulus control may help. Use the bed and bedroom only for sleep and sex. Wait until you are sleepy to go to bed. If unable to go to sleep in a reasonable time (for example, 15-20 minutes), get out of bed and leave the bedroom. Do something boring. Read a dull book. When sleepy, return to the bedroom and start the process over again. Get up at a fixed time in the morning. Do not nap during the day. For the first few days fatigue and tiredness during the day will be present. Slowly, sleep will improve in duration and quality.

The last technique which has been helpful is sleep restriction. With this technique, the amount of time allowed for sleep is reduced and fixed. Once sleeping well during the restricted time, the amount of time allowed for sleep is gradually extended until an optimal amount of time for sleep is reached.

When using sleep restriction, a fixed wake-up time and an estimate of the number of hours you usually sleep are needed to start. Someone who sleeps only four hours a night would be allowed only 4 1/4 hours to sleep on the first few nights of sleep restriction.

The wake-up time will be fixed and determines the time to end sleep. If the wake-up time is 6 A.M., then bedtime is 4 1/4 hours before, at 1:45 A.M.

The first few days of restricted sleep time will result in sleepiness and fatigue during the day. It is important not to take naps. Once the 4 1/4 hours allowed for sleep are mostly time asleep (90%), then the time to go to bed may be moved earlier by a quarter-hour. As each further night's sleep improves, an extra quarter-hour may be added to the time allowed to sleep. Gradually, the time for sleeping will increase to a length which results in better sleep. Each patient will find an appropriate time for his own condition.

Medications are available to assist sleep onset and sleep duration. They are used extensively in situations of short-term insomnia which occur in hospitals. While they offer a simple solution to short-term situations, they are not a solution for long-term insomnia. There are major problems with sleep medications when used for long periods of time. When used night after night, they become less effective and eventually stop working. They often affect the type and quality of sleep. The amount of sleep in some levels (stages) may be reduced or increased, and they often become habit-forming. After use for a number of months, sleep will not occur for several nights when the medication is stopped. In some situations, drug withdrawal symptoms may occur if the medication is stopped suddenly.

Medications may have a role in the treatment of chronic insomnia. They should be used with care and for a limited time. A physician can help you with your questions.

Conclusions

Chronic insomnia is a difficult problem for many individuals. There are no simple solutions, but professional advice may help you to achieve better sleep. The techniques described have helped many sleep longer and better. They are all interrelated. Personal habits, relaxation techniques and sleep restriction share many common principles. Incorporating these principles into your life can help. It is always helpful to remember that many famous people suffered from insomnia. Such notable individuals as Albert Schweitzer and Alexander Graham Bell are reported to have had difficulty with sleep. Yet, they were able to achieve many things and their accomplishments should inspire and reassure those with insomnia. Thomas Edison reportedly only slept six hours a day and has been quoted as saying, "Sleep is a waste of time". Difficulty sleeping may be a cause for concern, but certainly not a reason for inactivity or withdrawing from life.

Insomnia
CHAPTER SUMMARY

Insomnia — The symptoms of not sleeping well. The perception of not getting enough sleep. It is the difficulty going to sleep and staying asleep.

CAUSES OF INSOMNIA
➤ Personal Habits
—Excessive eating and drinking
—Using too much caffeine and alcohol
➤ Medical conditions — colds, pain or cancer
➤ Psychiatric illnesses — depression and schizophrenia
➤ Sleep disorders — sleep apnea, periodic limb movements
➤ Medications
➤ Anxiety and stress

PSYCHOPHYSIOLOGIC INSOMNIA
➤ Personal response to life and its difficulties
➤ The result of stress and emotional turmoil

(continued on next page)

Insomnia
CHAPTER SUMMARY (*continued*)

CHRONIC INSOMNIA
➤ Insomnia present for months or years
➤ May be a result of medical, psychiatric and sleep problems or their treatment
➤ No cause apparent — common situation
  —Triggering events not apparent
  —Insomnia becomes a part of lives
➤ Insomnia persists
  —Personal Habits
  —Working too hard at sleeping
  —Perception

TREATMENT OF CHRONIC INSOMNIA
➤ Goal of treatment — Improve the quality of sleep
➤ Reassurance
➤ Relaxation techniques
➤ Stimulus control techniques
➤ Sleep restriction techniques
➤ Medications

CONCLUSIONS
➤ Chronic insomnia — difficult problem
➤ Professional assistance valuable
➤ Many famous insomniacs

Chapter 13

Narcolepsy

Narcolepsy is a disorder of unknown cause which has been recognized by physicians for over one hundred years. Patients with narcolepsy have excessive daytime sleepiness and usually have sleep attacks. A striking feature in some individuals is sudden physical collapse. Narcolepsy usually begins before the age of 25 years in most cases, however, it can develop in people as old as fifty. Symptoms may take several years to develop and all may not be present in each individual with narcolepsy.

Narcolepsy will usually have its onset early in life. The disease will start with one or two symptoms and others may develop over several months or years. The disease is lifelong and its effects vary. For some, symptoms may be minor or well-controlled with medications. For others there may be periods of time when the symptoms are hard to control or treatment is less effective. Most individuals with narcolepsy can live normal lives but some have chronic problems from the disease.

SYMPTOMS

The symptoms of narcolepsy include excessive daytime sleepiness, irresistible sleep attacks, episodes of collapse or weakness (cataplexy), sleep paralysis, and sleep onset hallucinations. Some of these symptoms were once thought to be only seen with narcolepsy. Now it is known that they all may be associated with other sleep disorders with the exception of cataplexy.

Excessive daytime sleepiness

Often gradual in onset, increased sleepiness from narcolepsy occurs first in the afternoon. The sleepiness may progress to other parts of the day or remain limited to one portion of it. For most individuals who are known to have narcolepsy, the sleepiness can be very strong and affect their daytime activities.

Irresistible sleep attacks

Episodes of severe sleepiness occur with narcolepsy and are usually irresistible. They will come on during normal activities such as talking, eating, standing and walking. Most patients have two or three attacks per day. They may sleep from one to two minutes or up to twenty or more before awaking and feeling a little refreshed afterwards.

Napping

Frequent napping is often used by someone with narcolepsy to avoid sleep attacks and excessive sleepiness. The technique is effective many times in preventing some symptoms.

Cataplexy

Cataplexy is a specific symptom of narcolepsy. It is a sudden loss of muscle tone that can last from a few seconds to minutes. It can be minor or major, involve a few selected muscles or can result in weakness of the entire body. The person may have problems keeping the eyes open or just holding up the head or extremities. A more serious form of cataplexy would be a complete collapse to the floor. A person may either remain conscious with these attacks or have sleep. They are commonly brought on by strong emotions — laughter, anger, fear, surprise. Cataplexy may occur very infrequently, with an episode every few years. On the other hand, episodes can be as frequent as several times a day.

Sleep paralysis

Sleep paralysis refers to a problem that happens while falling asleep or waking up. When it occurs, the person feels an inability to move or speak although they are awake. They are able to breathe and move their eyes but nothing else. The episodes are usually brief, although they can last for up to 10 or 20 minutes. They can occur often or infrequently and be quite frightening.

Sleep-onset hallucinations

These events can be thought of as a dream mixed with a normal awareness when falling asleep. Before fully going to sleep, the visual events of the moment — actual location — become intermixed with a dreamlike experience. The dream portion can include almost any content but most frequently is visual with realistic content involving humans or animals. They are noted in about two-thirds of patients with narcolepsy and may occur once a year or daily. They can happen with sleep paralysis.

CAUSES

Narcolepsy is a disease of unknown cause. There is evidence that genetic factors are important. It is associated with certain gene types and it does occur in families.

The symptoms of narcolepsy can be caused by diseases of the brain. Brain tumors, multiple sclerosis, encephalitis, strokes and other problems have been shown to cause the symptoms of narcolepsy. Most of the symptoms can also be caused by other sleep disorders such as sleep apnea syndrome.

The disease, narcolepsy, is not associated with changes in the brain or nerves. There are no physical (anatomical) changes that have been identified. Rather, it is a problem of brain function, the nature of which has not been clearly established.

DIAGNOSIS

Most of the symptoms of narcolepsy can occur in other problems that cause excessive daytime sleepiness. Sleep-related symptoms should be reviewed carefully and a physical exam performed by a knowledgeable physician. Although sometimes a diagnosis may be established on this information, usually other causes of excessive daytime sleepiness must be excluded before a diagnosis of narcolepsy can be made.

Several tests are employed to confirm a diagnosis of narcolepsy. A sleep study will be performed to exclude other causes of disturbed sleep. Daytime sleepiness will be tested with a multiple sleep latency test. Blood may be drawn for genetic testing. Unfortunately, there is no specific test for narcolepsy. Only when the test results and the patient's history and physical exam demonstrate a typical picture, can a diagnosis be made.

TREATMENT

Narcolepsy is treated several ways. The approach to treatment can be divided into general measures and specific medications

General Measures

Many methods may be used to improve the quality of a person's sleep and lessen the effect of his narcolepsy. It is important that the sleep habits promote good sleep. Careful attention to promoting a restful night's sleep lessens the natural tendency to daytime sleepiness. Someone with narcolepsy has more difficulty with their daytime symptoms when their nights are not restful.

Any medical problems or other sleep problems that may cause excessive daytime sleepiness should be treated and controlled as much as possible. Just as poor sleep habits promote daytime sleepiness in normal persons and in those with narcolepsy, medical illness and other sleep problems such as sleep apnea cause added problems during the day. If a person with narcolepsy has significant additional problems, the narcolepsy will be much more difficult to control.

Daytime sleepiness can be helped with planned naps. If a person has problems falling asleep at several separate times during the day, taking short naps at planned times will help prevent the sleepiness and avoid accidents.

Medications

The symptoms of narcolepsy can be treated beneficially with medications. Specific agents can be used to treat the symptoms of excessive sleepiness and others to treat the symptoms of cataplexy. Each patient's program must be specifically designed for his symptoms. A knowledgeable physician must direct the use of medications and design a program to fit the patient.

Medications for excessive sleepiness have been used for many years as the main treatment for narcolepsy. They include the central nervous system stimulants such as Ritalin, Dexedrine, and Cylert. Provigil is a newer agent that promotes wakefulness without the side-effects of the stimulants. The dose needed and the agent of choice will vary with the person and physician.

Cataplexy does not improve on medications designed to treat excessive sleepiness. A separate group of drugs have been found to be helpful in the treatment of the cataplexy of narcolepsy. Interestingly, these drugs come from the agents used to treat depression that are known to affect the brain's biochemistry. Drugs include Tofranil, Anafranil, and Vivactil. The newer serotonin re-uptake inhibitors also can be used to treat cataplexy including Prozac, Paxil, and Zoloft. Like the drugs for sleepiness, the dose required and the medication chosen will depend upon the symptoms and the physician. Careful monitoring of the patient will be required till a satisfactory result is achieved.

Narcolepsy
CHAPTER SUMMARY

LIFE-LONG DISORDER OF EXCESSIVE SLEEPINESS

- Usual onset before age 25
- Progressive over several years
- Symptoms controlled with medications

SYMPTOMS

- Excessive daytime sleepiness
- Irresistible sleep attacks
- Cataplexy — Episodes of weakness
- Sleep onset hallucinations
- Sleep paralysis with sleep onset or awaking

CAUSE

- Unknown
- A tendency to run in families

DIAGNOSIS

- Symptoms may be caused by other diseases
- Symptoms may occur with other medical problems
- Diagnosis requires examination and testing by an experienced physician

(continued on next page)

Narcolepsy
CHAPTER SUMMARY *(continued)*

TREATMENT

➤ General

—Good sleep habits

—Prompt treatment of other medical and sleep disorders

➤ Medications for sleepiness

—Stimulants - Ritalin, Dexedrine, and Cylert

—Other - Provigil

➤ Medications for cataplexy - Antidepressants

—Tofranil, Anafranil and Vivactil

—Prozac, Paxil and Zoloft

➤ Excellent control of symptoms often achieved

Chapter 14

Legs and Sleeping— Periodic Limb Movements

There are a surprising number of individuals who have leg problems that can interrupt sleep or keep them from going to sleep. Three major types of problems can be identified. These are leg cramps, restless legs and periodic limb movements.

LEG CRAMPS

As we grow older, leg cramps often occur during sleep. They may be quite severe awakening you from sleep with the pain. Nocturnal leg cramps occur in normal healthy people as well as in those with certain medical conditions. In most cases, no reason for the cramps can be identified. They may occur after an overly active day, after a specific exercise involving the legs or for no apparent reason. Leg cramps can occur with circulatory and metabolic disorders. Your physician can help evaluate you for possible causes.

Leg cramps can often be easily treated. Two of the most common forms of treatment are vitamin E and quinine. Vitamin E taken as a supplement often eliminates leg cramps. Four-hundred units a day is the most common dose. Quinine comes in various forms. It is available over-the-counter as a tablet. Quinine water is widely available as "tonic water". An eight-ounce glass of tonic water a day will often cure leg cramps.

RESTLESS LEGS

There are people who experience problems with their legs as they try to go to sleep. They may have feelings of irritation, tingling or just the need to move their legs. In a severe form, the legs may actually jerk as they try to relax. These symptoms are called restless legs or restless legs syndrome.

Restless legs symptoms may occur without a recognized medical problem. But more commonly, they are seen in association with a large number of medical disorders, usually metabolic and circulatory. Congestive heart failure, renal failure, and iron deficiency are the most common medical conditions that lead to restless legs. However, there are many others. Sometimes periodic limb movement disorder can be present with the restless legs symptoms.

The treatment of restless legs is usually directed at improving the associated medical illness or at controlling the symptoms. Symptomatic treatment suppresses the movements and allows for better sleep, but it is temporary. It will not correct the underlying problem.

PERIODIC LIMB MOVEMENTS (MYOCLONUS)

Brief, uncontrolled spasms of the leg and arm muscles when going to sleep and while asleep sometimes occur. They may be strong enough to shake the bed, or they may be weak, not seen and recorded only with sensitive electrical instruments. When these spasms occur repeatedly, they are called "periodic limb movements." In the past, the term "myoclonus" was used to describe this problem.

In many individuals, periodic limb movements are present and do not cause a problem. They may be observed by a spouse or someone watching the person sleep. Although alarming, if sleep is not disturbed, they are of no significance. Commonly, they are recognized on a sleep study where a recording of leg muscle activity is obtained.

On the other hand, periodic limb movements can cause problems, even serious ones. The spasms become important when sleep is affected. If a significant percentage of the spasms causes the patient to arouse or awake from sleep, a problem may be present. Repeated awakenings disrupt sleep and result in daytime fatigue and sleepiness. Repeated movements at sleep onset may make getting to sleep difficult and result in the complaints of insomnia.

Periodic limb movements may be seen with many medical conditions and with other sleep problems such as sleep apnea. When that occurs, treating those problems often results in clearing up the periodic limb movements.

Treating periodic limb movements not secondary to another medical problem can be difficult. A number of prescribed drugs have been used. Your physician can help you choose an appropriate treatment.

Legs and Sleeping
Periodic Limb Movements
CHAPTER SUMMARY

LEG CRAMPS
- Muscle spasms in calves
- Usually no medical reason
- Seen in circulatory and metabolic disorders
- Treatments
  - —Vitamin E
  - —Quinine

RESTLESS LEGS
- A feeling of irritation, tingling or uneasiness
- A need to move the legs
- Commonly seen in people with congestive heart failure, renal failure and iron deficiency
- Treatment directed at the associated conditions along with suppressing the sensations and the need to move

PERIODIC LIMB MOVEMENTS
- Uncontrolled muscle jerks of legs or arms
- Varies from weak to strong
- May prevent or delay sleep onset — causes insomnia
- May disturb or interrupt sleep — causes daytime sleepiness
- Often associated with other medical problems
- Treatment available but difficult

Chapter 15

Jet Lag

More often now than ever before, we are traveling and working around the world. The advent of commercial passenger jets has led to a revolution in the speed and distance we travel. Jet lag has become a well-known problem following trips crossing several time zones.

Why do we get jet lag? What is it? Jet lag occurs when our body has need for sleep and rest at the wrong time. After we travel rapidly to a different time and place, the sun, the clock and our plans say it is time to act. But, our bodies want to rest and sleep. After traveling to a new time zone, our bodies want to do what they have always done when they have always done it.

Sleep and the Circadian Rhythm

Jet lag is the most common problem experienced with the effect of our biologic rhythm, the circadian rhythm, on sleep. The circadian rhythm is the biological clock in our brains that controls many functions of

139

our bodies. Hormone levels, body temperature and a host of other things change in relation to the time of day. Sleep and wakefulness are under the strong influence of the rhythm. While the effects can be overcome, it requires considerable effort to resist the natural tendency the rhythm promotes.

Sleep is required to provide time for the body to rest and rebuild for new activity, for a new day. In normal situations, the rhythm encourages sleep onset at the same time every day. The clock runs on a 24-hour cycle, repeating it each day. There are situations in which a person's clock runs on a time other than 24-hours that can lead to significant problems. Other situations change the time during the day we need to work and sleep. A change of work hours from day to night will shift the time we need to be alert and the time available for sleep. Traveling over several time zones also has the same effect.

Feelings of exhaustion and a need for sleep grow stronger as we approach our normal sleep schedule. We feel bright and alert in the day as we go about our activities. We may only be aware of these feelings when our activities change and we stay up later or get up earlier than normal. The circadian rhythm has a momentum that is fixed and hidden in our daily routines. While going about these routines, the strong effects of the rhythm fit into our lives as we give into its wishes.

The rhythm follows a certain pattern and has phases for being awake and asleep. The body's clock appears to be set by the effect of sunlight on the eyes. The exact mechanism is unclear but bright light encourages the biological clock to start the rhythm of biological functions on their 24-hour cycle. Changing the eyes' exposure to light will change what the body's clock wants you to do and when you are to do it.

Travel and Sleep

Mankind has divided the world into time zones as a practical way to handle the changes in daytime and nighttime across the earth. When it is noon in New York City and the sun is directly overhead, the sun appears low in the morning sky in Los Angeles. Time zones adjust the local clock time to the daily appearance of the sun — making it noon when it should be noon.

When we travel over long distances, we pass through many time zones. It is not unusual for international travelers to pass through six, eight or even twelve time zones during a single journey. For example, traveling from New York to Paris you will pass through six time zones. Going from Chicago to New Delhi, India, you will travel halfway around the world and cross twelve time zones. Often this travel occurs rapidly. The six to twelve time zones may be crossed in less than twenty-four hours. Jet lag symptoms are worse after eastward rather than westward flights, increase with the number of time zones crossed, and are more intense in the older person.

Remember the momentum of the circadian rhythm. After traveling to our new location, our bodies want to sleep at the same time we slept at home. If it is 10 P.M. (our bedtime) at home, we will want to sleep even if it is 10 A.M. where we have traveled. Our rhythm affects how we feel and our need for sleep whether we travel over twelve time zones or two.

Compensating for Time Zone Changes

We sleep because we need to restore our fatigued bodies and because our bodies believe it is time to sleep. Our

PLANNING FOR JET LAG

➤ What direction will you be traveling?

➤ What is the time difference between your home and your destination?

➤ Can you adjust your schedule before leaving for your new destination?

➤ Will your air travel be overnight?

➤ How many hours of sleep can you get on the airplane?

➤ What time of the day will you arrive at your new location?

➤ Will you have an opportunity to rest on arrival?

➤ What activities can you do before your planned first night of sleep?

➤ What is your planned bedtime at the new location?

activities dictate the degree of fatigue present and our biological clock tells us whether it is time to sleep. Both of these factors must be considered when trying to overcome jet lag. We must try to take care of both our exhaustion and our clock.

Fortunately our bodies will adjust to the new time zone gradually, because of the effect of light on our circadian rhythm. It requires several days for these changes to occur and for you to adapt to the new time. Meanwhile, you will feel irritable, out of sorts, and sleepy or alert at the wrong times. There may be difficulties concentrating, fatigue, disorientation or light-headedness. Stomach problems may be present. When you travel for work or even for pleasure, the length of your stay may not allow you to enjoy or get the most from your trip because of jet lag. However, with some planning, the period required to adjust to the new time zone can be shortened.

Planning and adjusting can begin days before the trip. The number of zones crossed, the duration of the journey, the direction of the travel and the number of days you will be at the new location should all be considered. When planning, remember that it is easier to travel from east to west. In addition, it is always easier to delay sleep onset rather than force yourself to sleep earlier.

There is some scientific evidence that the use of sleep aids may help establish a new sleep schedule when traveling. Both prescription sleep medications and over-the-counter agents such as melatonin have been suggested as treatments which may speed adjustment to new time zones. They may help with the onset of sleep at the new desired sleep time or with napping during a long flight. When used on a temporary basis, they promote sleep onset and help establish a new cycle or rhythm at a time when it may be difficult to go to sleep.

Efforts to adjust your cycle may begin by changing your home routine. The time you sleep at home can be adjusted somewhat a few days before departure by getting up early or going to bed later in anticipation of the time for sleep at your new location. Traveling overseas usually involves an extended air flight, often at night. The opportunity to sleep during the flight should be taken and planned as part of the day's rest.

The day of arrival at the new location will be day one of a new time zone. Always plan to rest when traveling. We need to rest to counteract the exhaustion brought on by the work and stress of travel to a strange and possibly exotic location. But, we should try to get as much of our rest as possible at the time for sleep in our new location.

When we arrive exhausted at midday in Europe after an almost sleepless overnight flight from the United States, we feel the intense need to sleep and to rest. It is alright to rest, but try to keep it a brief nap and be careful not to sleep away the day. It is important to get out into the daylight as soon and as much as possible.

For your first day in Europe, try to stay up until a normal bedtime before retiring for the night. You should be really tired by that time, and you should sleep. Don't be surprised if you wake in the middle of the night or very

REDUCING JET LAG

GOALS FOR TRAVEL

➤ Sleep as much as possible during the flight.

➤ Use alcohol and caffeine as little as possible during the flight.

➤ Nap as little as possible during the day at your destination.

➤ Try to follow a fixed bedtime and rising time at your destination.

➤ Enjoy the experience and your trip. Jet lag is part of modern travel.

early in the morning. Resist the urge to start the day at three or four in the morning. It is best to try to sleep or rest till your normal morning waking time.

Your second day in Europe should see you out in the daylight as soon as possible. Just as the nap on arrival pays back some of your exhaustion debt, the effect of the light of day on your biological clock is equally important. For several days you will feel excessive fatigue during the day. Be ready and plan for rest periods, but stick to your bedtime and awaking time.

Light, probably along with other environmental clues, serves as a stimulation to our biological clocks. It will actually adjust and reset them. It will take a few days before a new setting becomes fully adjusted. The most important step is getting you and your eyes out into the light of day — morning light.

Jet Lag
CHAPTER SUMMARY

Jet lag is the feeling we experience when we travel to a new location several time zones from our home. Symptoms of inappropriate sleepiness, irritability, light-headedness, stomach problems and insomnia may occur.

SLEEP AND THE CIRCADIAN RHYTHM
➤ Sleep is controlled by a biological clock.
➤ The Circadian Rhythm is the name of the biological clock.
➤ The strong effects of the rhythm are hidden in our daily lives.

(continued on next page)

Jet Lag
CHAPTER SUMMARY *(continued)*

Sleep and the Circadian Rhythm (continued)

➤ The rhythm has a strong momentum.
➤ The rhythm is primarily controlled by light with the help of other environmental factors.

TRAVEL AND SLEEP

➤ Time zones were created by man to relate the position of the sun with the earth.
➤ Modern travel can move us through many time zones rapidly.
➤ After travel, our circadian rhythm wants us to sleep when we slept at home.
➤ Jet lag is the result of our rhythm being out of cycle with our location and activities.

COMPENSATING FOR TIME ZONE CHANGES

➤ Plan ahead.
➤ Adjust your sleep schedule before leaving.
➤ Sleep while you travel.
➤ Do not sleep during the day at your destination.
➤ Establish a fixed bedtime and arising time at your destination.
➤ During the day, get out into the daylight as soon as possible.

SECTION V

APPENDICES

This section includes some useful additional information for those who wish to pursue their problems and questions further.

How to Sleep Well

Epworth Sleepiness Scale

Sleep Diary

Additional Readings

Web Sites

Organizations

Glossary

Index

Section V — Appendices

HOW TO SLEEP WELL

Things to Do:

—Go to bed at the same time every night

—Get out of bed at the same time each morning

—Exercise regularly

—Make the bedroom as dark, comfortable, and quiet as possible

Hints:

—Only use your bedroom for sleep and sex

—Pay attention to how you feel in the morning

—Note how much sleep is required for you to feel rested

—Have a pre-sleep ritual / Repeat same steps daily

Naps:

—Only take naps if you sleep well at night

—If you take a nap, do it in the afternoon

—Keep naps as short as possible

If You Can't Sleep:

—Do not lie awake in bed for long periods of time

—If you can't fall asleep within 20 minutes

   - Get out of bed and do something relaxing

   - Return to bed when sleepy and try again

(continued on next page)

HOW TO SLEEP WELL
(continued)

Avoid:

—Eating heavy or spicy meals in the evening

—Eating late meals

—Drinking large quantities of liquid late in the evening

—Exercising vigorously in the evening

—Eating or watching television in bed

—Drinking caffeinated beverages late in the day

THE EPWORTH SLEEPINESS SCALE*

This is a test you may take on your own to estimate your sleepiness. A total score of less than 10 is normal. Scores over 15 suggest an excessive level of sleepiness.

How likely are you to doze off or fall asleep in the following situations, in contrast to feeling just tired? This refers to your usual way of life in recent times. Even if you have not done some of these things recently, try to work out how they would have affected you. Use the following scale to choose the most appropriate number for each situation:

> 0 = would never doze
>
> 1 = slight chance of dozing
>
> 2 = moderate chance of dozing
>
> 3 = high chance of dozing

* Sleep, 14(6):540-545,1991

Appendix - The Epworth Sleepiness Scale

SITUATION	CHANCE OF DOZING
Sitting and reading	_____
Watching TV	_____
Sitting, inactive in a public place (e.g. a theater or a meeting)	_____
As a passenger in a car for an hour without a break	_____
Lying down to rest in the afternoon when circumstances permit	_____
Sitting and talking to someone	_____
Sitting quietly after lunch without alcohol	_____
In a car, while stopped for a few minutes in traffic	_____

Sleep Diary

SLEEP DIARY
What you need to know

Purpose: A sleep diary can help identify reasons for having problems sleeping. It can help you understand your sleep problem by recording daily patterns. It is an excellent way to inform your physician of your sleep history.

How it works: A daily record is kept of sleep and activities related to sleep. After recording a daily diary for five or more days, the information is reviewed for patterns which suggest causes for disturbed sleep.

When to start: If you are having a problem, start this evening. The daily diary begins each day at bedtime and ends at bedtime the next day. No preparation is required. Only a pen and the diary are needed.

Events of importance: There are many events and activities which affect sleep quality. It is impossible to record them all. The purpose of the diary is to look for patterns. While details may be important, the diary should be used to show the big picture of your life.

153

The details will be requested later by your physician if he feels they are needed. The following information will be helpful for the diary: time in bed; time asleep; nap times; exercise; meals; smoking; alcohol; caffeine or chocolate intake; and medications taken.

How to record the information:
— Start tonight.
— Plan to record information twice a day. The best times are on arising and at bedtime.
— Put tonight's date on the first page.
— Complete the first section in the morning.
— Complete the next section at the end of your day.
— Provide your best estimate of time. It is impossible to know exactly the times involved.
— If you are unsure of the answer to a question, just note it with a question mark.

Evaluating your sleep diary: There are two ways to evaluate your sleep diary. Just reviewing the daily information may be helpful. Or, the information may be charted to be more easily reviewed.

USING A SLEEP DIARY

➤ A record of your sleep pattern and habits
➤ A record of one day of your life
➤ Begins when you go to bed for the night
➤ Ends when you go to bed the next night
➤ Use the questionnaire, or chart, or both

Sleep Diary Questionnaire

NAME:_____ DATE:_____

ANSWER AND COMPLETE IN THE MORNING UPON AWAKENING

Time in bed for the night: _____

How long were you in bed before you went to sleep last night?

_____ minutes or _____ hours

What time did you get out of bed for the day? _____

How was your night's sleep? _____ good _____ fair _____ poor

Are you sleepy now? ___ Yes ___ No

Did you wake up during the night? ___ No *** Skip to next question

___ Yes *** How many times?   1   2   3   4   5   or more

*** Complete the information below

* *

Episode	How long awake?	Reason*
1	_____	_____
2	_____	_____
3	_____	_____
4	_____	_____

*Reason examples — bathroom, noise, sweats, choking, dreams, no reason, cannot remember

* *

Have you done the following since going to bed?

Taken medications? ___ No ___ Yes

Please list at what times taken _____,_____,_____,_____

Drunk alcohol? ___ No ___ Yes

Times? _____,_____,_____,_____,_____

Drunk beverages containing caffeine? ___ No ___ Yes

Times? _____,_____,_____,_____,_____

Eaten snacks? ___ No ___ Yes

Time of snacks? _____,_____,_____,_____,_____

Eaten meals? ___ No ___ Yes

Time? _____ Small, Medium or Large

Time? _____ Small, Medium or Large

Exercised? ___ No ___ Yes

Time? _____ Duration _____ Mild, Moderate, or Heavy

(continued on next page)

SLEEP DIARY QUESTIONNAIRE (continued)

ANSWER AND COMPLETE AT BEDTIME

Are you sleepy now? ___ No ___ Yes

Did you take a nap since getting out of bed for the day? ___ No
___ Yes ***How many times? 1 2 3 4 5 or more
***Complete the information below

****

Nap Episode	How long asleep?	Reason*
1		
2		
3		
4		

*Reason examples — always do, tired, bored, sleepy,
no reason, cannot remember

****

Have you done the following since getting out of bed for the day?

Taken medications? ___ No ___ Yes
Times? _____,_____,_____,_____

Drunk alcohol? ___ No ___ Yes
Times? _____,_____,_____,_____,_____

Drunk beverages containing caffeine? ___ No ___ Yes
Times? _____,_____,_____,_____,_____

Eaten snacks? ___ No ___ Yes
Times? _____,_____,_____,_____,_____

Eaten meals? ___ No ___ Yes
Time? _____ Small, Medium or Large
Time? _____ Small, Medium or Large
Time? _____ Small, Medium or Large
Time? _____ Small, Medium or Large

Exercised? ___ No ___ Yes
Time? _____ Duration _____ Mild, Moderate, or Heavy
Time? _____ Duration _____ Mild, Moderate, or Heavy

Time in bed for the night: _____

Are you sleepy? ___ No ___ Yes

Did you take any medications at bedtime? ___ No ___ Yes

Did you take any sleeping aids at bedtime? ___ No ___ Yes

Sleep Diary

Date of night started: _____   Time started (bedtime): _____   Time completed (bedtime next day): _____

(Instructions: Use the abbreviations below in the appropriate box to indicate time event occurred)

Diary Time

Events:

Time started (S)
Time completed (C)

Time in bed (X-X)
Time asleep (As-As)
Naps out of bed (Np)

Meals (M)
Snacks (S)
Caffeine (C)
Alcohol (A)
Medications (Rx)

Exercise (E)

Notes: _____

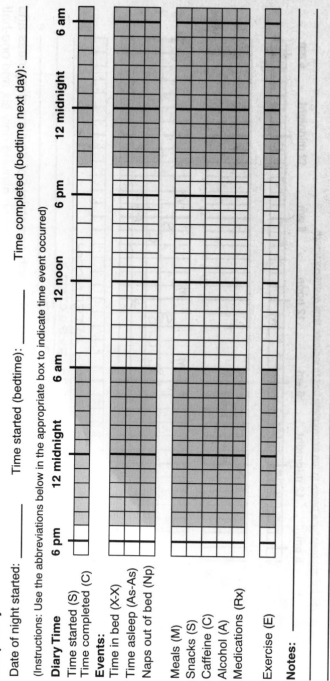

Figure Appendix -1

Sleep Diary

Date of night started: Dec 9, 1999 Time started (bedtime): 11:30 PM Time completed (bedtime next day): 11:15 PM

(Instructions: Use the abbreviations below in the appropriate box to indicate time event occurred)

Diary Time	6 pm	12 midnight	6 am	12 noon	6 pm	12 midnight	6 am

Time started (S)
Time completed (C)

Events:

Time in bed (X-X)
Time asleep (As-As)
Naps out of bed (Np)

Meals (M)
Snacks (S)
Caffeine (C)
Alcohol (A)
Medications (Rx)

Exercise (E)

Notes: TIRED IN MORNING AND EARLY AFTERNOON

NO MEDICATIONS   NO EXERCISE

HEARTBURN AT 3AM + 4:30 AM

This is an example of a sleep diary from a 55 year old male with complaints of daytime sleepiness and tiredness. It gives a sample of how the diary may be filled out. This person allowed only six and one-half hours for sleep. His sleep was interrupted by heartburn twice. During the day he used a significant amount of caffeine and alcohol both of which may contribute to heartburn and poor sleep.   Figure Appendix -2

RECOMMENDED READING

General

SLEEP: EVERYTHING YOU NEED TO KNOW
by J. Paul Caldwell, M.D.

Firefly Books LTD: 1997. This is a well organized book which strengths are coverage of non sleep apnea subjects.

ALL I WANT IS A GOOD NIGHT'S SLEEP
by Sonia Ancoli-Israel

Mosby: 1996. The major strengths of this book are in areas other than sleep apnea.

COMPLETE IDIOTS GUIDE TO GETTING A GOOD NIGHT'S SLEEP, THE
by Martin Moore-Ede, M.D. and Susanne LeVert

Alpha Books: 1998. This is a very complete, well illustrated book.

SLEEP - THE GENTLE TYRANT
by Wilse B. Webb

Anker Publishing Company, Inc.: 1992. This book covers the subject of sleep in detail including normal and abnormal sleep.

Sleep Apnea

PHANTOM OF THE NIGHT: OVERCOME SLEEP
APNEA SYNDROME AND SNORING - WIN YOUR
HIDDEN STRUGGLE TO BREATHE, SLEEP AND LIVE
by T. Scott Johnson, M.D. and Jerry Halberstadt

New Technology Publishing, Inc.: 1992. The most comprehensive book for those who suffer from sleep apnea. It is detailed and full of information.

Snoring

THE SNORING CURE : SIMPLE STEPS TO GETTING
A GOOD NIGHT'S SLEEP
by Laurence A. Smolley M.D. and Debra Fulghum Bruce

W. W. Norton and Company: 1999. Snoring is the focus of this volume.

SNORING FROM A TO ZZZ
by Derek S. Lipman B.D.
Spencer Press. 1998. Focuses on the symptom of snoring.

WEB SITES OF VALUE

The number of internet sites grows and changes daily. The following sites are good starting points for the internet user. They provide valuable information and refer to many interesting additional sites.

http://www.asda.org This is the site of the American Academy of Sleep Medicine. This location can provide links to many additional locations with valuable information about sleep and its disorders.

http.//www.sleepnet. com This site is also valuable as a starting point for investigating sleep on the web.

http.//www.sleepfoundation.org This is an excellent site for basic general information on sleep disorders and their treatments.

http.//www.sleepapnea.org The American Sleep Apnea Association is an organization for patients and professionals concerned with sleep apnea and its consequences.

http.//www.narcolepsynetwork.org This site is hosted by the Narcolepsy Network, an organization that concentrates its efforts on narcolepsy.

http.//www.rls.org The Restless Legs Syndrome Foundation is the host of this site which provides an excellent starting point for those with Restless Legs Syndrome.

ORGANIZATIONS

American Sleep Apnea Association - An organization directing its attention to sleep apnea, education and awareness, research and improvements in care.

> American Sleep Apnea Association
> 1424 K. Street NW, Suite 302
> Washington, D.C 20005
> http://www.sleepapnea.org

National Sleep Foundation - This independent foundation is dedicated to improving public health through the understanding of sleep and sleep disorders.

National Sleep Foundation
1522 K Street NW, Suite 500
Washington, D.C. 20005
http://www.sleepfoundation.org

Narcolepsy Network - This is an organization whose membership consists of those who suffer from narcolepsy, their families and friends, and professionals with an interest in the disease.

Narcolepsy Network
10921 Reed Hartman Highway
Cincinnati, OH 45242
http://www.narcolepsynetwork.org

Restless Legs Syndrome Foundation - This group focuses its attention and efforts on the Restless Legs Syndrome and its effects.

RLS Foundation
819 Second Street SW
Rochester, Minnesota
http://www.rls.org

GLOSSARY

A

Advanced sleep phase syndrome - A disorder characterized by normal sleep which begins and ends sooner than desired.

Alzheimer's Disease - A common form of dementia characterized by memory problems, confusion, and loss of mental capacity. The cause is unknown.

Antibiotics - A class of drugs used in the treatment of infections which kill or antagonize bacteria.

Antidepressants - A class of drugs used in the treatment of depression.

Antihistamines -A class of drugs which antagonize the effects of histamine and are used in the treatment of allergies.

Apnea - The term applied to an absence of breathing for a period of 10 seconds or longer.

Apnea index - The average number of apneas which occur during an hour of sleep.

Arousal - An event during sleep characterized by going from deeper sleep to lighter sleep without awakening.

164 • *Sleep and its Disorders*

B

Bi-level CPAP - A form of Nasal CPAP which has pressures that change with inspiration and expiration.

Benign - A term which indicates a favorable situation, outcome or prognosis. A benign tumor is not malignant.

C

Cataplexy - A sudden loss of muscle tone which can result in partial weakness or collapse of the entire body. The episodes can last for minutes. Cataplexy is usually associated with a diagnosis of narcolepsy.

Central sleep apnea - Sleep apnea caused by a failure to breathe. No breathing occurs because the brain does not tell the chest to move. Central sleep apnea accounts for less than 1% of sleep apnea problems.

Chronic insomnia - The insomnia for which no cause is apparent after study and which has been present for months or years.

Circadian rhythm - The rhythmic changes in physiology that occur within the human body. These changes are usually associated with a 24-hour cycle of the day and night and consist of regular changes in metabolic functions. They are controlled by a portion of the brain.

Confusional arousals - Episodes of confusion or disorientation occurring upon awaking.

Constant Positive Airway Pressure (CPAP) - A medical technique to supply air under pressure to the nose, mouth, pharynx, larynx and tracheobronchial tree.

D

Delayed sleep phase syndrome - A disorder characterized by normal sleep which has both its onset and ending later than desired.

Duration (of sleep) -The duration of sleep is the time from sleep onset to the final awakening in the morning prior to getting out of bed.

E

Electrocardiogram (ECG or EKG) - The electrocardiogram is a measurement of the electrical activity of the heart. By placement of sensitive electrodes on the skin, the electrical activity generated by the heart can be measured and recorded.

Electroencephalogram (EEG) - The EEG is a measurement of electrical activity of the brain. It is performed by placing sensitive electrodes on the skin of the scalp to measure the electrical activity generated by the brain. This technique is used to measure the presence of sleep, the depth of sleep, the change in sleep pattern and is essential to measuring sleep architecture.

EEG (See electroencephalogram)

Electromyogram (EMG) - The electromyogram is a measurement of the electrical activity in muscles generated by muscular contractions. It is performed by placing sensitive electrodes on specific muscles.

Electro-oculogram (EOG) - The electro-oculogram measures eye movements by monitoring small changes in electrical activity through sensitive electrodes placed on the skin near the eye.

EMG (See electromyogram)

EOG (See electro-oculogram)

F

Fiberoptic -A type of flexible glass tube which allows for transmission of light. Fiberoptic tubes allow for viewing of internal body organs.

H

Hygiene (sleep) (See sleep hygiene)

Hypnic jerk - A sudden muscular jerk which occurs while falling asleep. This is a normal event and is commonly experienced.

Hypopnea -A decrease in breathing which causes one or more changes in oxygen, breathing effort or sleep stage. It is usually caused by a partial airway obstruction.

Hypopnea index - The number of hypopneas occurring during an hour of sleep.

I

Idiopathic Obstructive Sleep Apnea Syndrome - Sleep apnea syndrome that results from upper airway obstruction of unknown cause.

Insomnia -Insomnia is the term applied to the problems of going to sleep, staying asleep or getting enough sleep at night.

J

Jet lag - The temporary disruption of the sleep and wake cycles caused by rapid travel through several time zones.

L

Laryngoscopy - Looking at the pharynx and larynx through an instrument. Usually an examination performed with the aid of fiberoptic tubes.

Larynx - The larynx is located at the upper portion of the trachea and at the bottom of the pharynx. It is commonly known as the voice box and serves as the entryway into the trachea. It is the organ of speech where the vocal cords are located.

LAUP (Laser-Assisted Uvulopalatoplasty) - A surgical procedure using a laser to remove a portion of the soft palate.

M

Mandible - The lower jawbone.

Maxilla - The upper jawbone which forms the hard palate and floor of the nasal cavity.

MSLT (multiple sleep latency test) - A test used to measure sleepiness. A recording of brain wave activity is made during repeated daytime naps.

Multiple sleep latency test (See MSLT)

Myoclonus - Older term, now replaced by periodic leg movements.

N

Narcolepsy - A disease with the primary symptoms of excessive daytime sleepiness associated with irresistible sleep attacks.

Nasal CPAP - The application of positive airway pressure through a mask applied to the nose. A common form of treatment for sleep apnea.

Neurologist - A specialist in the diseases of the neuromuscular system, often trained or experienced in the treating of disorders of sleep.

Night terrors - Shouting, thrashing, kicking or other some-times violent active behaviors during sleep. Night terrors is one of the parasomnias.

Non REM sleep - All stages of sleep other than REM sleep.

O

Obstructive sleep apnea - Sleep apnea caused by obstruction of the airway during sleep.

Oropharynx (See pharynx)

Otolaryngologist - A specialist in the diseases and surgical treatment of the ears, nose and throat, often trained or experienced in the treatment of disorders of sleep.

Oxygen - An element found in gas form which is essential for life.

Oxygen saturation - The amount of oxygen carried in the blood as a percentage of the amount possible. A 90% oxygen saturation or greater is considered an adequate amount of oxygen.

P

Palate - A plate of bone and tissue separating the lower portion of the nose from the upper portion of the mouth.

Parasomnias - The group of diseases associated with movement or activity during sleep.

Periodic limb movements - Rapid muscular contractions of the legs, and occasionally arms, during sleep. Although usually not visible, they can interrupt sleep and cause problems.

Pharynx - The common space where the mouth and nose meet and connect to the larynx and esophagus. It is separated into the nasopharynx, oropharynx and hypopharynx.

Polysomnogram (See sleep studies)

Presleep ritual - A pattern of activity repeated each night before sleep.

Psychiatrist - A physician specializing in the diagnosis and treatment of mental disorders.

Psychophysiologic (insomnia) - A classification for disorders resulting from the stresses and anxieties of life and a person's reactions to those events.

Pulmonary hypertension - A form of high blood pressure which is limited to the arterial blood vessels in the lungs (pulmonary arteries).

Pulmonologist - A specialist in diseases of the thorax and breathing. Often trained or experienced in treating disorders of sleep.

R

REM (rapid eye movement sleep) - A sleep stage where the closed eyes move rapidly, the body's muscles are totally relaxed and the brain appears to be awake. This stage is often associated with dreaming.

REM Behavior Disorder - A disorder characterized by physical behavior such as walking, shouting or thrashing which occurs during REM sleep.

Restless legs - The term applied to an irritability of the legs, improved by movement, which occurs when trying to go to sleep at night.

Rheumatoid Arthritis - A chronic systemic disease which affects many tissues throughout the body but primarily the joints of the hands and feet.

Rhythmic Movement Disorder - A disorder characterized by repetitive unusual movement at the onset of sleep.

S

Schizophrenia - A mental illness characterized by components of delusions, hallucinations, disordered speech and behavior, blunted emotional responses and mental deterioration.

Shift work - Term applied to working hours of the day other than the traditional morning and afternoon time.

Sleep apnea - The occurrence of apnea during sleep.

Sleep apnea syndrome - The association of abnormal sleep caused by apneas or hypopneas and symptoms and signs caused by the disturbed sleep.

Sleep architecture - This is the term that is used to describe brain wave patterns during sleep. In order to determine sleep architectures, measurements must be made of brain waves (EEG), muscular activities (EMG) and eye movements (EOG).

Sleep diary - A personal record of sleep and awake activities and the habits which affect sleep.

Sleep duration (See Duration)

Sleep habits - Personal behavior which affects the quality and quantity of sleep.

Sleep hygiene - Our personal habits which affect sleep quality.

Sleep paralysis - The feeling of not being able to move that occurs while going to sleep and awakening from sleep. This may be a normal phenomenon or seen with sleep disorders.

Sleep specialist - A person who by training or experience is knowledgeable about the disorders of sleep and cares for and advises patients with sleep problems.

Sleep stage - A distinctive pattern of brain waves (EEG), muscular activity (EMG) and eye movements (EOG). These patterns are defined according to criteria for each of these measurements and can be used to measure the type of sleep that has occurred.

Sleep study - A continuous recording of physiologic variables during sleep which include brain waves (EEG), muscle tones (EMG), eye movements (EOG), respirations, heart rhythm, oxygen saturation and airflow at the nose and mouth.

Sleep talking - Talking during sleep.

Sleep terrors - A condition in which activity occurs during sleep that suggests a person is experiencing a frightening event.

Sleepwalking - The activity, while asleep, of walking, climbing or moving about.

Snoring - The noise made by vibration of the soft palate and uvula during sleep. Snoring usually indicates some upper airway narrowing.

Soft palate - The portion of the palate at the back of the throat which contains no supporting bone.

Stimulus control therapy - A technique used to treat some forms of psychological insomnia in which the bedroom is used for only sleep and sex.

T

Tonsillectomy - A surgical procedure to remove the tonsils.

Tonsils - Lymphatic tissue located in the oral pharynx at the base of the soft palate on each side of the throat.

Trachea - The air tube which connects the lungs with the larynx.

Tracheostomy - A surgical procedure to create an opening in the upper neck to the trachea.

U

Upper Airway Resistance - Obstructive events that occur during sleep without a significant drop in airflow or oxygen level but which result in an arousal from sleep. When these events occur often, the symptoms of sleep apnea syndrome appear.

Uvula - Tissue which hangs down from the back of the soft palate.

Uvulopalatopharyngoplasty - A surgical procedure which is used to treat obstructive sleep apnea and consists of removing tissue from the palate and pharynx.

Uvulopalatoplasty - A surgical procedure used to treat snoring in which tissue is removed from the soft palate.

INDEX

Index

Parasomnias - 51-55
Periodic limb movements -
36, 42, 137
Pharynx - 63-66
Polysomnogram - 18-22, 82,
84
Psychiatrists - 16
Psychophysiologic insomnia
- 34, 118
Pulmonary hypertension -
81
Pulmonologist - 16

R

REM (rapid eye movement
sleep) - 8, 10
REM Behavior disorders - 54
Restless legs - 37, 136
Rhythmic movement disor-
der - 53

S

Shift Work - 46
Sleep, Normal - 1, 5-8, 69,
111
Duration - 6, 12, 33, 39
Time - 7, 45-48, 110
Movements during - 51
Environment - 110
Sleep apnea - 59-61, 67, 70
Central - See central
sleep apnea
Idiopathic - 78, 79, 91
Positional - 86, 93
Temporary - 85

Sleep apnea syndrome - 61,
73
Causes - 77-79
Complications - 81-83
Signs - 75
Symptoms - 74
Severity - 83-84, 89
Test for - 82
Treatment - 89-105
Sleep architecture - 8, 11
Sleep diary - 16, 153
Sleep disordered breathing -
40, 59-61
Sleep hygiene (habits) - see
Habits
Sleep laboratory - 18-21
Sleep paralysis - 129
Sleep restriction therapy -
123
Sleep specialist - 16
Sleep stages - 8, 60
Sleep study - 18-22
Sleepiness - 42, 43
excessive - 39, 82, 84
Sleep talking - 53
Sleep terrors - 52, 54
Sleepwalking - 52
Snoring - 67, 70, 75, 85, 101
Soft palate - 62, 65, 66
Stimulus control therapy -
123

T

Throat - 63-66
Tonsils - 63-66, 77, 80